Competency Based
Logbook of
General Medicine

Compiled for all Phases of MBBS

Designed as per the latest CBME Curriculum for Indian Medical Graduate

Student's Name: _____

Roll No. _____   Year/Session: _____

Name of the Institution: _____

Name of the University: _____

Competency Based
Logbook of
General Medicine

Compiled for all Phases of MBBS

Designed as per the latest CBME Curriculum for Indian Medical Graduate

Neeraj Mahajan MD, DNB, ACME
Co-Convenor, NMC Nodal Center for Faculty Development
Associate Professor of Physiology
Smt. NHL Municipal Medical College
Ahmedabad, Gujarat

Paras Parekh MD (Gold Medal), ACME Fellow
MEU Coordinator for Faculty Development
Professor of Physiology
Gujarat Adani Institute of Medical Sciences,
Bhuj, Gujarat

Chanchal Shrivastav PhD, ACME Fellow
MEU Co-Coordinator for Faculty Development
Professor of Physiology
Ananta Institute of Medical Sciences & Research Center
Rajsamand, Rajasthan

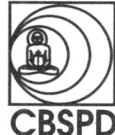

CBSPD

CBS Publishers & Distributors Pvt Ltd

New Delhi • Bengaluru • Chennai • Kochi • Kolkata • Lucknow • Mumbai
Hyderabad • Jharkhand • Nagpur • Patna • Pune • Uttarakhand

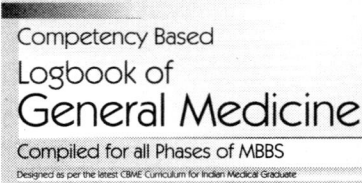

Competency Based
Logbook of
General Medicine
Compiled for all Phases of MBBS
Designed as per the latest CBME Curriculum for Indian Medical Graduate

ISBN: 978-93-90709-64-9

Copyright © Authors and Publisher

First Edition: 2021
Reprint 2022, 2024 **2025**

Published by Satish Kumar Jain and produced by Varun Jain for
CBS Publishers & Distributors Pvt Ltd
4819/XI Prahlad Street, 24 Ansari Road, Daryaganj, New Delhi 110 002, India
Ph: 011-23289259, 23266861   e-mail: delhi@cbspd.com   Website: www.cbspd.com

Corporate Office: 204 FIE, Industrial Area, Patparganj, Delhi 110 092, India
Ph: 011-49344934   Fax: 011-49344935   e-mail: publishing@cbspd.com; publicity@cbspd.com

Branches

- **Bengaluru:** Seema House 2975, 17th Cross, K.R. Road, Banasankari 2nd Stage, Bengaluru 560 070, Karnataka, India
  Ph: +91-80-26771678/79   Fax: +91-80-26771680   e-mail: bangalore@cbspd.com
- **Chennai:** 7, Subbaraya Street, Shenoy Nagar, Chennai 600 030, Tamil Nadu, India
  Ph: +91-44-26680620, 26681266   Fax: +91-44-42032115   e-mail: chennai@cbspd.com
- **Kochi:** 42/1325, 1326, Power House Road, Opposite KSEB, Power House, Ernakulum 682 018, Kochi, Kerala, India
  Ph: +91-484-4059061–67   Fax: +91-484-4059065   e-mail: kochi@cbspd.com
- **Kolkata:** 147, Hind Ceramics Compound, 1st Floor, Nilgunj Road, Belghoria, Kolkata 700 056, West Bengal, India
  Ph: +91-33-25330055/56   e-mail: kolkata@cbspd.com
- **Lucknow:** Basement, Khushuma Complex, 7 Meerabai Marg (behind Jawahar Bhawan), Lucknow 226 001, UP, India
  Ph: +91-522-4000032   e-mail: tiwari.lucknow@cbspd.com
- **Mumbai:** PWD Shed, Gala No. 25/26, Ramchandra Bhatt Marg, Next JJ Hospital Gate No. 2, Opp. Union Bank of India,
  Noorbaug, Mumbai 400 009, Maharashtra, India
  Ph: +91-22-66661880/89   e-mail: mumbai@cbspd.com

Representatives

• **Hyderabad**	0-9885175004	• **Jharkhand**	0-9811541605	• **Nagpur**	0-8692091830
• **Patna**	0-9334159340	• **Pune**	0-9923910676	• **Uttarakhand**	0-9716462459

Printed at: SRK Graphics, Delhi, India.

Preface

This *Logbook of General Medicine* is structured longitudinally to record all the activities of learner from 2nd professional to 3rd professional part II of MBBS. Pages for AETCOM Modules, Pandemic module, Skill training and Seminar presentation also included in this logbook as per the guidelines of Competency Based Medical Education (CBME) Curriculum.

All psychomotor and affective domain competencies are printed in this Logbook but faculty/department has flexibility to priorities these further. For each competency, longitudinal activities done by learner across all the phases of MBBS can be recorded on a same page so that it becomes easier to assess the progress of learner.

This Logbook will also serve the role of learner's portfolio as provision for reflective writing is also there.

Hope this Logbook will aid in the journey of becoming competent Indian Medical Graduate (IMG).

Best wishes....

Neeraj Mahajan
Paras Parekh
Chanchal Shrivastav

Guidelines to use this Logbook

Logbook is a verified record of the progression of the learner documenting the acqusition of the requisite knowledge, skills, attitude and/ or competencies.[1] Successful documentation and submission of the logbook is a prerequisite for being allowed to take the final summative examination (GMER 11.1.1.b.7).[2]

This compiled Logbook of General Medicine is designed to be used across all phases of MBBS.

What is included in this Logbook?

1. Competencies which need to be certified

2. All 'show how' level competencies in psychomotor and communication domain

3. Provision to record activities related to AETCOM module, pandemic module, skill training, and seminar presentation

4. Provision for the reflective writing to benefit students to become an active, aware and critical learner.

> *Note: Selection of competencies to record in Logbook is at the discrete of faculty/department.*

Explanation of the Logbook Table

✖ **Name of activity:** Predefined task to be performed by learner to achieve stated objective or competency. (Note: Multiple sessions may be required for the acquisition of a single objective or competency)

✖ **Phase description with date of completion:** Name of phase along with date of completion of activity (e.g. Phase III part I, dd-mm-yyyy)

✖ **Attempt:** Objective achieved in
  ✧ First **(F)** attempt or
  ✧ Repeat **(R)** attempt or
  ✧ Remedial **(Re)** attempt

> *Note: Remedial (Re) is a planned activity to rectify the mistakes or problems faced by the learner in achieving the intended outcome.*

✖ **Rating:** The faculty will assess the performance level of learner whether it is
  ✧ Satisfactory **(Meets expectations 'M')** or
  ✧ Need improvement **(Below expectation 'B')**

Guidelines to use this Logbook

- **Decision of faculty:** The faculty will decide and mark the status of activity as
  - ✧ **Completed (C)** if objective is achieved or
  - ✧ **Not completed (NC)** if repeat or remedial attempt is given
- Initial (Signature) of faculty indicating the completion or other determination
- Initial (Signature) of the learner if feedback has been received

Example 1: How to document if objective is achieved in first attempt

	IM 1.18/ IM 8.17: Perform & Interpret 12 Lead ECG (Note: Learner need to achieve this competency 3 times individually)						
S No.	Name of Activity	Phase description with date of completion	Attempt First (F) Repeat (R) Remedial (Re)	Rating below Expectation (B) Meet Expectation (M)	Decision of Faculty Completed (C) Not Completed (NC)	Faculty Initial with date	Feedback received Initial of learner
1.	Placing ECG leads properly	Phase III Part I 11/12/2020	F	M	C		

Example 2: How to document if objective is achieved in repeat attempt

	IM 1.18/ IM 8.17: Perform & Interpret 12 Lead ECG Note: Learner need to achieve this competency 3 times individually)						
S No.	Name of Activity	Phase Description with Date of Completion	Attempt First (F) Repeat (R) Remedial (Re)	Rating Below Expectation (B) Meet Expectation (M)	Decision of Faculty Completed (C) Not Completed (NC)	Faculty Initial with Date	Feedback Received Initial of Learner
1.	Placing ECG leads properly	Phase III Part I 11/12/2020	F	B	NC		Repeat the activity
2.	Placing ECG leads properly	Phase III Part I 14/12/2020	R	M	C		

Example 3: How to document if objective is achieved in remedial attempt

<table>
<tr><td colspan="8">IM 1.18/ IM 8.17: Perform & Interpret 12 Lead ECG
(Note: Learner need to achieve this competency 3 times individually)</td></tr>
<tr>
<td>S No.</td>
<td>Name of Activity</td>
<td>Phase Description with
Date of Completion</td>
<td>Attempt
First (F)
Repeat (R)
Remedial (Re)</td>
<td>Rating
Below Expectation (B)
Meet Expectation (M)</td>
<td>Decision of Faculty
Completed (C)
Not Completed (NC)</td>
<td>Faculty Initial with Date</td>
<td>Feedback Received
Initial of Learner</td>
</tr>
<tr>
<td>1.</td>
<td>Placing ECG leads properly</td>
<td>Phase III Part I 11/12/2020</td>
<td>F</td>
<td>B</td>
<td>NC</td>
<td></td>
<td>Repeat the activity</td>
</tr>
<tr>
<td>2.</td>
<td>Placing ECG leads properly</td>
<td>Phase III Part I 14/12/2020</td>
<td>R</td>
<td>B</td>
<td>NC</td>
<td></td>
<td>Planning of Remedial Session</td>
</tr>
<tr>
<td>3.</td>
<td>Placing ECG leads properly</td>
<td>Phase III Part I 17/12/2020</td>
<td>Re</td>
<td>M</td>
<td>C</td>
<td></td>
<td></td>
</tr>
</table>

For AETCOM module and Pandemic module, please refer respective document available on website of National Medical Commission (NMC).

References

1. Logbook guidelines document dated 17.01.2020.
2. Graduate Medical Education Regulation document dated 06.11.2019.

Guidelines for Reflective Writing

Reflection is a personal response to any new information or experience which enhances critical thinking and learning. Reflective writing is a very powerful tool for teaching-learning and assessment of affective domain.

How to write Reflection

Reflection is written under following three headings.

What happened?

1. What was the session & who conducted it?

So what?

2. What key points did I take away from the sessions?
3. What interested and motivated me about these sessions?
4. What were new skills and information or understanding for me?
5. Describe holistic learning (skill, attitude, knowledge, communication, emotional, psychological, all)
6. Why I learned what I learned and why I can't learn what I can't learned?
7. How I learned best? (Learning style)
8. Include both good and bad points and why
9. Include both professional and personal gains

What next?

10. How will I use this learning for the benefit of society and will this learning shape me up into a better doctor? Then what ideas I should use immediately and which ones, better for future application?

Reflective writing is based on Gibbs and Kolb's reflective learning cycle: AAAA

Any Experience
↓
Affect / Feelings (both good and bad)
↓
Analyse, theorise and conclude the learning
↓
Action plan for future

Certificate of completion

This is to certify that the candidate Mr./Ms. _____

Son/Daughter of _____admitted in the year 20___ - 20___ at the

_____ has satisfactorily completed/has not

completed all assignments/requirements mentioned in the Logbook for MBBS course in the subject

of General Medicine. He / She is / is not eligible to appear for the University examination.

Head of the Department
Date:

University Enrollment No.:

Competency Based Logbook of General Medicine

Clinical Posting Completions			
	Date of Posting	*Name of Unit*	*Signature of Head of the Unit*
Clinical Posting 1			
Clinical Posting 2			
Clinical Posting 3			
Clinical Posting 4			
Clinical Posting 5			
Clinical Posting 6			

Student Profile

Name of Student: _____

Date of Birth: _____

MBBS Batch: _____

Blood Group: _____

| Paste Passport size |
| Photograph here |

Student's Mobile No: _____

Student's E-mail id: _____

Parents Details:

Father's Name: _____

Mobile No: _____

Occupation: _____

Mother's Name: _____

Mobile No: _____

Occupation: _____

Present Address: _____

Permanent Address: _____

_____

_____

Signature of the Student

Contents

CERTIFIABLE COMPETENCIES

Certifiable Competencies

IM 1.18/ IM 8.17: Perform & Interpret 12 Lead ECG
(Note: Learner need to achieve this competency 3 times individually)

S No.	Name of Activity	Phase Description with Date of Completion	Attempt First (F) Repeat (R) Remedial (Re)	Rating Below Expectation (B) Meet Expectation (M)	Decision of Faculty Completed (C) Not Completed (NC)	Faculty Initial with Date	Feedback Received Initial of Learner

Certifiable Competencies							
IM 2.10: Order, Perform & Interpret an ECG **(Note: Learner need to achieve this competency 3 times individually)**							
S No.	Name of Activity	Phase Description with Date of Completion	Attempt First (F) Repeat (R) Remedial (Re)	Rating Below Expectation (B) Meet Expectation (M)	Decision of Faculty Completed (C) Not Completed (NC)	Faculty Initial with Date	Feedback Received Initial of Learner

Certifiable Competencies

IM 2.22: Perform and demonstrate in a mannequin BLS
(Note: Learner need to achieve this competency once individually)

S No.	Name of Activity	Phase Description with Date of Completion	Attempt First (F) Repeat (R) Remedial (Re)	Rating Below Expectation (B) Meet Expectation (M)	Decision of Faculty Completed (C) Not Completed (NC)	Faculty Initial with Date	Feedback Received Initial of Learner

	Certifiable Competencies						
IM 11.12: Perform and interpret a capillary blood glucose test **(Note: Learner need to achieve this competency 2 times individually)**							
S No.	Name of Activity	Phase Description with Date of Completion	Attempt First (F) Repeat (R) Remedial (Re)	Rating Below Expectation (B) Meet Expectation (M)	Decision of Faculty Completed (C) Not Completed (NC)	Faculty Initial with Date	Feedback Received Initial of Learner

Certifiable Competencies

IM 11.13: Perform and interpret a urinary ketone estimation with a dipstick
(Note: Learner need to achieve this competency 2 times individually)

S No.	Name of Activity	Phase Description with Date of Completion	Attempt First (F) Repeat (R) Remedial (Re)	Rating Below Expectation (B) Meet Expectation (M)	Decision of Faculty Completed (C) Not Completed (NC)	Faculty Initial with Date	Feedback Received Initial of Learner

GENERAL COMPETENCIES (SHOW HOW LEVEL)

Topic 1: Heart Failure							
S. No.	Name of Activity	Phase Description with Date of Completion	Attempt First (F) Repeat (R) Remedial (Re)	Rating Below Expectation (B) Meet Expectation (M)	Decision of Faculty Completed (C) Not Completed (NC)	Faculty Initial with Date	Feedback Received Initial of Learner
IM 1.10: Elicit document and present an appropriate history that will establish the diagnosis, cause and severity of heart failure including: presenting complaints, precipitating and exacerbating factors, risk factors exercise tolerance, changes in sleep patterns, features suggestive of infective endocarditis							

S. No.	Name of Activity	Phase Description with Date of Completion	Attempt First (F) Repeat (R) Remedial (Re)	Rating Below Expectation (B) Meet Expectation (M)	Decision of Faculty Completed (C) Not Completed (NC)	Faculty Initial with Date	Feedback Received Initial of Learner
Topic 1: Heart Failure							
IM 1.11: Perform and demonstrate a systematic examination based on the history that will help establish the diagnosis and estimate its severity including: measurement of pulse, blood pressure and respiratory rate, jugular venous forms & pulses, peripheral pulses, conjunctiva and fundus, lung, cardiac examination including palpation and auscultation with identification of heart sounds and murmurs, abdominal distension and splenic palpation							

Topic 1: Heart Failure							
S. No.	Name of Activity	Phase Description with Date of Completion	Attempt First (F) Repeat (R) Remedial (Re)	Rating Below Expectation (B) Meet Expectation (M)	Decision of Faculty Completed (C) Not Completed (NC)	Faculty Initial with Date	Feedback Received Initial of Learner
IM 1.11: Perform and demonstrate a systematic examination based on the history that will help establish the diagnosis and estimate its severity including: measurement of pulse, blood pressure and respiratory rate, jugular venous forms & pulses, peripheral pulses, conjunctiva and fundus, lung, cardiac examination including palpation and auscultation with identification of heart sounds and murmurs, abdominal distension and splenic palpation							

Topic 1: Heart Failure							
S. No.	Name of Activity	Phase Description with Date of Completion	Attempt First (F) Repeat (R) Remedial (Re)	Rating Below Expectation (B) Meet Expectation (M)	Decision of Faculty Completed (C) Not Completed (NC)	Faculty Initial with Date	Feedback Received Initial of Learner
IM 1.12: Demonstrate peripheral pulse, volume, character, quality and variation in various causes of heart failure							

Topic 1: Heart Failure							
S. No.	Name of Activity	Phase Description with Date of Completion	Attempt First (F) Repeat (R) Remedial (Re)	Rating Below Expectation (B) Meet Expectation (M)	Decision of Faculty Completed (C) Not Completed (NC)	Faculty Initial with Date	Feedback Received Initial of Learner
IM 1.13: Measure the blood pressure accurately, recognize and discuss alterations in blood pressure in valvular heart disease and other causes of heart failure and cardiac tamponade							

S. No.	Name of Activity	Phase Description with Date of Completion	Attempt First (F) Repeat (R) Remedial (Re)	Rating Below Expectation (B) Meet Expectation (M)	Decision of Faculty Completed (C) Not Completed (NC)	Faculty Initial with Date	Feedback Received Initial of Learner
Topic 1: Heart Failure							
IM 1.14: Demonstrate and measure jugular venous distension							

S. No.	Name of Activity	Phase Description with Date of Completion	Attempt First (F) Repeat (R) Remedial (Re)	Rating Below Expectation (B) Meet Expectation (M)	Decision of Faculty Completed (C) Not Completed (NC)	Faculty Initial with Date	Feedback Received Initial of Learner
IM 1.15: Identify and describe the timing, pitch quality conduction and significance of precordial murmurs and their variations							

Topic 1: Heart Failure

Topic 1: Heart Failure							
S. No.	Name of Activity	Phase Description with Date of Completion	Attempt First (F) Repeat (R) Remedial (Re)	Rating Below Expectation (B) Meet Expectation (M)	Decision of Faculty Completed (C) Not Completed (NC)	Faculty Initial with Date	Feedback Received Initial of Learner
IM 1.17: Order and interpret diagnostic testing based on the clinical diagnosis including 12 lead ECG, Chest radiograph, blood cultures							

General Competencies (Show How Level)

S. No.	Name of Activity	Phase Description with Date of Completion	Attempt First (F) Repeat (R) Remedial (Re)	Rating Below Expectation (B) Meet Expectation (M)	Decision of Faculty Completed (C) Not Completed (NC)	Faculty Initial with Date	Feedback Received Initial of Learner
Topic 1: Heart Failure							
IM 1.20: Determine the severity of valvular heart disease based on the clinical and laboratory and imaging features and determine the level of intervention required including surgery							

19

S. No.	Name of Activity	Phase Description with Date of Completion	Attempt First (F) Repeat (R) Remedial (Re)	Rating Below Expectation (B) Meet Expectation (M)	Decision of Faculty Completed (C) Not Completed (NC)	Faculty Initial with Date	Feedback Received Initial of Learner
Topic 1: Heart Failure							

IM 1.21: Describe and discuss and identify the clinical features of acute and subacute endocarditis, echocardiographic findings, blood culture and sensitivity and therapy

Topic 1: Heart Failure							
S. No.	Name of Activity	Phase Description with Date of Completion	Attempt First (F) Repeat (R) Remedial (Re)	Rating Below Expectation (B) Meet Expectation (M)	Decision of Faculty Completed (C) Not Completed (NC)	Faculty Initial with Date	Feedback Received Initial of Learner
IM 1.22: Assist and demonstrate the proper technique in collecting specimen for blood culture							

Topic 1: Heart Failure							
S. No.	**Name of Activity**	**Phase Description with Date of Completion**	**Attempt First (F) Repeat (R) Remedial (Re)**	**Rating Below Expectation (B) Meet Expectation (M)**	**Decision of Faculty Completed (C) Not Completed (NC)**	**Faculty Initial with Date**	**Feedback Received Initial of Learner**
IM 1.23: Describe, prescribe and communicate non pharmacologic management of heart failure including sodium restriction, physical activity and limitations							

S. No.	Name of Activity	Phase Description with Date of Completion	Attempt First (F) Repeat (R) Remedial (Re)	Rating Below Expectation (B) Meet Expectation (M)	Decision of Faculty Completed (C) Not Completed (NC)	Faculty Initial with Date	Feedback Received Initial of Learner
Topic 1: Heart Failure							

IM 1.26: Develop document and present a management plan for patients with heart failure based on type of failure, underlying aetiology

S. No.	Name of Activity	Phase Description with Date of Completion	Attempt First (F) Repeat (R) Remedial (Re)	Rating Below Expectation (B) Meet Expectation (M)	Decision of Faculty Completed (C) Not Completed (NC)	Faculty Initial with Date	Feedback Received Initial of Learner

Topic 1: Heart Failure							
S. No.	Name of Activity	Phase Description with Date of Completion	Attempt First (F) Repeat (R) Remedial (Re)	Rating Below Expectation (B) Meet Expectation (M)	Decision of Faculty Completed (C) Not Completed (NC)	Faculty Initial with Date	Feedback Received Initial of Learner
IM 1.30: Administer an intramuscular injection with an appropriate explanation to the patient							

Topic 2: Ischemic Heart Disease

S. No.	Name of Activity	Phase Description with Date of Completion	Attempt First (F) Repeat (R) Remedial (Re)	Rating Below Expectation (B) Meet Expectation (M)	Decision of Faculty Completed (C) Not Completed (NC)	Faculty Initial with Date	Feedback Received Initial of Learner
IM 2.6: Elicit document and present an appropriate history that includes onset evolution, presentation risk factors, family history, comorbid conditions, complications, medication, history of atherosclerosis, IHD and coronary syndromes							

S. No.	Name of Activity	Phase Description with Date of Completion	Attempt First (F) Repeat (R) Remedial (Re)	Rating Below Expectation (B) Meet Expectation (M)	Decision of Faculty Completed (C) Not Completed (NC)	Faculty Initial with Date	Feedback Received Initial of Learner
Topic 2: Ischemic Heart Disease							
IM 2.7: Perform, demonstrate and document a physical examination including a vascular and cardiac examination that is appropriate for the clinical presentation							

S. No.	Name of Activity	Phase Description with Date of Completion	Attempt First (F) Repeat (R) Remedial (Re)	Rating Below Expectation (B) Meet Expectation (M)	Decision of Faculty Completed (C) Not Completed (NC)	Faculty Initial with Date	Feedback Received Initial of Learner
IM 2.8: Generate document and present a differential diagnosis based on the clinical presentation and priorities based on "cannot miss", most likely diagnosis and severity							

Topic 2: Ischemic Heart Disease

	Topic 2: Ischemic Heart Disease						
S. No.	Name of Activity	Phase Description with Date of Completion	Attempt First (F) Repeat (R) Remedial (Re)	Rating Below Expectation (B) Meet Expectation (M)	Decision of Faculty Completed (C) Not Completed (NC)	Faculty Initial with Date	Feedback Received Initial of Learner
IM 2.9: Distinguish and differentiate between stable and unstable angina and AMI based on the clinical presentation							

	Topic 2: Ischemic Heart Disease						
S. No.	Name of Activity	Phase Description with Date of Completion	Attempt First (F) Repeat (R) Remedial (Re)	Rating Below Expectation (B) Meet Expectation (M)	Decision of Faculty Completed (C) Not Completed (NC)	Faculty Initial with Date	Feedback Received Initial of Learner
IM 2.11: Order and interpret a Chest X-ray and markers of acute myocardial infarction							

S. No.	Name of Activity	Phase Description with Date of Completion	Attempt First (F) Repeat (R) Remedial (Re)	Rating Below Expectation (B) Meet Expectation (M)	Decision of Faculty Completed (C) Not Completed (NC)	Faculty Initial with Date	Feedback Received Initial of Learner
Topic 2: Ischemic Heart Disease							
IM 2.12: Choose and interpret a lipid profile and identify the desirable lipid profile in the clinical context							

Topic 2: Ischemic Heart Disease							
S. No.	Name of Activity	Phase Description with Date of Completion	Attempt First (F) Repeat (R) Remedial (Re)	Rating Below Expectation (B) Meet Expectation (M)	Decision of Faculty Completed (C) Not Completed (NC)	Faculty Initial with Date	Feedback Received Initial of Learner
IM 2.24: Counsel and communicate to patients with empathy lifestyle changes in atherosclerosis / post coronary syndromes							

S. No.	Name of Activity	Phase Description with Date of Completion	Attempt First (F) Repeat (R) Remedial (Re)	Rating Below Expectation (B) Meet Expectation (M)	Decision of Faculty Completed (C) Not Completed (NC)	Faculty Initial with Date	Feedback Received Initial of Learner
Topic 3: Pneumonia							
IM 3.4: Elicit document and present an appropriate history including the evolution, risk factors including immune status and occupational risk							

	Topic 3: Pneumonia						
S. No.	Name of Activity	Phase Description with Date of Completion	Attempt First (F) Repeat (R) Remedial (Re)	Rating Below Expectation (B) Meet Expectation (M)	Decision of Faculty Completed (C) Not Completed (NC)	Faculty Initial with Date	Feedback Received Initial of Learner
M 3.5: Perform, document and demonstrate a physical examination including general examination and appropriate examination of the lungs that establishes the diagnosis, complications and severity of disease							

Topic 3: Pneumonia							
S. No.	Name of Activity	Phase Description with Date of Completion	Attempt First (F) Repeat (R) Remedial (Re)	Rating Below Expectation (B) Meet Expectation (M)	Decision of Faculty Completed (C) Not Completed (NC)	Faculty Initial with Date	Feedback Received Initial of Learner
IM 3.6: Generate document and present a differential diagnosis based on the clinical features, and priorities the diagnosis based on the presentation							

Topic 3: Pneumonia							
S. No.	Name of Activity	Phase Description with Date of Completion	Attempt First (F) Repeat (R) Remedial (Re)	Rating Below Expectation (B) Meet Expectation (M)	Decision of Faculty Completed (C) Not Completed (NC)	Faculty Initial with Date	Feedback Received Initial of Learner
IM 3.7: Order and interpret diagnostic tests based on the clinical presentation including: CBC, Chest X ray PA view, Mantoux, sputum gram stain, sputum culture and sensitivity, pleural fluid examination and culture, HIV testing and ABG							

Topic 3: Pneumonia							
S. No.	Name of Activity	Phase Description with Date of Completion	Attempt First (F) Repeat (R) Remedial (Re)	Rating Below Expectation (B) Meet Expectation (M)	Decision of Faculty Completed (C) Not Completed (NC)	Faculty Initial with Date	Feedback Received Initial of Learner
IM 3.8: Demonstrate in a mannequin and interpret results of an arterial blood gas examination							

S. No.	Name of Activity	Phase Description with Date of Completion	Attempt First (F) Repeat (R) Remedial (Re)	Rating Below Expectation (B) Meet Expectation (M)	Decision of Faculty Completed (C) Not Completed (NC)	Faculty Initial with Date	Feedback Received Initial of Learner
Topic 3: Pneumonia							
IM 3.9: Demonstrate in a mannequin and interpret results of a pleural fluid aspiration							

S. No.	Name of Activity	Phase Description with Date of Completion	Attempt First (F) Repeat (R) Remedial (Re)	Rating Below Expectation (B) Meet Expectation (M)	Decision of Faculty Completed (C) Not Completed (NC)	Faculty Initial with Date	Feedback Received Initial of Learner
Topic 3: Pneumonia							
IM 3.10: Demonstrate the correct technique in a mannequin and interpret results of a blood culture							

Topic 3: Pneumonia							
S. No.	Name of Activity	Phase Description with Date of Completion	Attempt First (F) Repeat (R) Remedial (Re)	Rating Below Expectation (B) Meet Expectation (M)	Decision of Faculty Completed (C) Not Completed (NC)	Faculty Initial with Date	Feedback Received Initial of Learner
IM 3.11: Describe and enumerate the indications for further testing including HRCT, Viral cultures, PCR and specialized testing							

S. No.	Name of Activity	Phase Description with Date of Completion	Attempt First (F) Repeat (R) Remedial (Re)	Rating Below Expectation (B) Meet Expectation (M)	Decision of Faculty Completed (C) Not Completed (NC)	Faculty Initial with Date	Feedback Received Initial of Learner
Topic 3: Pneumonia							
IM 3.12: Select, describe and prescribe based on the most likely aetiology, an appropriate empirical antimicrobial based on the pharmacology and antimicrobial spectrum							

S. No.	Name of Activity	Phase Description with Date of Completion	Attempt First (F) Repeat (R) Remedial (Re)	Rating Below Expectation (B) Meet Expectation (M)	Decision of Faculty Completed (C) Not Completed (NC)	Faculty Initial with Date	Feedback Received Initial of Learner
Topic 3: Pneumonia							
IM 3.13: Select, describe and prescribe based on culture and sensitivity appropriate empirical antimicrobial based on the pharmacology and antimicrobial spectrum							

		Topic 3: Pneumonia					
S. No.	Name of Activity	Phase Description with Date of Completion	Attempt First (F) Repeat (R) Remedial (Re)	Rating Below Expectation (B) Meet Expectation (M)	Decision of Faculty Completed (C) Not Completed (NC)	Faculty Initial with Date	Feedback Received Initial of Learner
IM 3.14: Perform and interpret a sputum gram stain and AFB							

Topic 3: Pneumonia						
S. No.	**Name of Activity**	**Phase Description with Date of Completion**	**Attempt First (F) Repeat (R) Remedial (Re)**	**Rating Below Expectation (B) Meet Expectation (M)**	**Decision of Faculty Completed (C) Not Completed (NC)**	**Faculty Initial with Date**	**Feedback Received** **Initial of Learner**
IM 3.18: Communicate and counsel patient on family on the diagnosis and therapy of pneumonia							

S. No.	Name of Activity	Phase Description with Date of Completion	Attempt First (F) Repeat (R) Remedial (Re)	Rating Below Expectation (B) Meet Expectation (M)	Decision of Faculty Completed (C) Not Completed (NC)	Faculty Initial with Date	Feedback Received Initial of Learner
Topic 4: Fever and febrile syndromes							
IM 4.9: Elicit document and present a medical history that helps delineate the aetiology of fever that includes the evolution and pattern of fever, associated symptoms, immune status, comorbidities, risk factors, exposure through occupation, travel and environment and medication use							

Topic 4: Fever and febrile syndromes							
S. No.	Name of Activity	Phase Description with Date of Completion	Attempt First (F) Repeat (R) Remedial (Re)	Rating Below Expectation (B) Meet Expectation (M)	Decision of Faculty Completed (C) Not Completed (NC)	Faculty Initial with Date	Feedback Received Initial of Learner
IM 4.10: Perform a systematic examination that establishes the diagnosis and severity of presentation that includes: general skin mucosal and lymph node examination, chest and abdominal examination (including examination of the liver and spleen)							

S. No.	Name of Activity	Phase Description with Date of Completion	Attempt First (F) Repeat (R) Remedial (Re)	Rating Below Expectation (B) Meet Expectation (M)	Decision of Faculty Completed (C) Not Completed (NC)	Faculty Initial with Date	Feedback Received Initial of Learner
	**IM 4.11: Generate a differential diagnosis and priorities based on clinical features that help distinguish between infective, inflammatory, malignant and rheumatologic causes**						

Topic 4: Fever and febrile syndromes

Topic 4: Fever and febrile syndromes

S. No.	Name of Activity	Phase Description with Date of Completion	Attempt First (F) Repeat (R) Remedial (Re)	Rating Below Expectation (B) Meet Expectation (M)	Decision of Faculty Completed (C) Not Completed (NC)	Faculty Initial with Date	Feedback Received Initial of Learner
IM 4.12: Order and interpret diagnostic tests based on the differential diagnosis including: CBC with differential, peripheral smear, urinary analysis with sediment, Chest X ray, blood and urine cultures, sputum gram stain and cultures, sputum AFB and cultures, CSF analysis, pleural and body fluid analysis, stool routine & culture and QBC							

	Topic 4: Fever and febrile syndromes						
S. No.	Name of Activity	Phase Description with Date of Completion	Attempt First (F) Repeat (R) Remedial (Re)	Rating Below Expectation (B) Meet Expectation (M)	Decision of Faculty Completed (C) Not Completed (NC)	Faculty Initial with Date	Feedback Received Initial of Learner
IM 4.13: Perform and interpret a sputum gram stain							

S. No.	Name of Activity	Phase Description with Date of Completion	Attempt First (F) Repeat (R) Remedial (Re)	Rating Below Expectation (B) Meet Expectation (M)	Decision of Faculty Completed (C) Not Completed (NC)	Faculty Initial with Date	Feedback Received Initial of Learner
IM 4.14: Perform and interpret a sputum AFB							

Topic 4: Fever and febrile syndromes							
S. No.	**Name of Activity**	**Phase Description with Date of Completion**	**Attempt First (F) Repeat (R) Remedial (Re)**	**Rating Below Expectation (B) Meet Expectation (M)**	**Decision of Faculty Completed (C) Not Completed (NC)**	**Faculty Initial with Date**	**Feedback Received Initial of Learner**
IM 4.15: Perform and interpret a malarial smear							

S. No.	Name of Activity	Phase Description with Date of Completion	Attempt First (F) Repeat (R) Remedial (Re)	Rating Below Expectation (B) Meet Expectation (M)	Decision of Faculty Completed (C) Not Completed (NC)	Faculty Initial with Date	Feedback Received Initial of Learner
Topic 4: Fever and febrile syndromes							
IM 4.17: Observe and assist in the performance of a bone marrow aspiration and biopsy in a simulated environment							

S. No.	Name of Activity	Phase Description with Date of Completion	Attempt First (F) Repeat (R) Remedial (Re)	Rating Below Expectation (B) Meet Expectation (M)	Decision of Faculty Completed (C) Not Completed (NC)	Faculty Initial with Date	Feedback Received Initial of Learner
Topic 4: Fever and febrile syndromes							
IM 4.19: Assist in the collection of blood and wound cultures							

S. No.	Name of Activity	Phase Description with Date of Completion	Attempt First (F) Repeat (R) Remedial (Re)	Rating Below Expectation (B) Meet Expectation (M)	Decision of Faculty Completed (C) Not Completed (NC)	Faculty Initial with Date	Feedback Received Initial of Learner
Topic 4: Fever and febrile syndromes							
IM 4.20: Interpret a PPD (Mantoux)							

S. No.	Name of Activity	Phase Description with Date of Completion	Attempt First (F) Repeat (R) Remedial (Re)	Rating Below Expectation (B) Meet Expectation (M)	Decision of Faculty Completed (C) Not Completed (NC)	Faculty Initial with Date	Feedback Received Initial of Learner
Topic 4: Fever and febrile syndromes							
IM 4.23: Prescribe drugs for malaria based on the species identified, prevalence of drug resistance and national programs							

Topic 4: Fever and febrile syndromes							
S. No.	Name of Activity	Phase Description with Date of Completion	Attempt First (F) Repeat (R) Remedial (Re)	Rating Below Expectation (B) Meet Expectation (M)	Decision of Faculty Completed (C) Not Completed (NC)	Faculty Initial with Date	Feedback Received Initial of Learner
IM 4.24: Develop an appropriate empiric treatment plan based on the patient's clinical and immune status pending definitive diagnosis							

S. No.	Name of Activity	Phase Description with Date of Completion	Attempt First (F) Repeat (R) Remedial (Re)	Rating Below Expectation (B) Meet Expectation (M)	Decision of Faculty Completed (C) Not Completed (NC)	Faculty Initial with Date	Feedback Received Initial of Learner
Topic 4: Fever and febrile syndromes							
IM 4.25: Communicate to the patient and family the diagnosis and treatment							

S. No.	Name of Activity	Phase Description with Date of Completion	Attempt First (F) Repeat (R) Remedial (Re)	Rating Below Expectation (B) Meet Expectation (M)	Decision of Faculty Completed (C) Not Completed (NC)	Faculty Initial with Date	Feedback Received Initial of Learner
Topic 4: Fever and febrile syndromes							
IM 4.26: Counsel the patient on malarial prevention							

Topic 5: Liver disease

S. No.	Name of Activity	Phase Description with Date of Completion	Attempt First (F) Repeat (R) Remedial (Re)	Rating Below Expectation (B) Meet Expectation (M)	Decision of Faculty Completed (C) Not Completed (NC)	Faculty Initial with Date	Feedback Received Initial of Learner
IM 5.9: Elicit document and present a medical history that helps delineate the aetiology of the current presentation and includes clinical presentation, risk factors, drug use, sexual history, vaccination history and family history							

Topic 5: Liver disease

S. No.	Name of Activity	Phase Description with Date of Completion	Attempt First (F) Repeat (R) Remedial (Re)	Rating Below Expectation (B) Meet Expectation (M)	Decision of Faculty Completed (C) Not Completed (NC)	Faculty Initial with Date	Feedback Received Initial of Learner
IM 5.10: Perform a systematic examination that establishes the diagnosis and severity that includes nutritional status, mental status, jaundice, abdominal distension ascites, features of portosystemic hypertension and hepatic encephalopathy							

General Competencies (Show How Level)

S. No.	Name of Activity	Phase Description with Date of Completion	Attempt First (F) Repeat (R) Remedial (Re)	Rating Below Expectation (B) Meet Expectation (M)	Decision of Faculty Completed (C) Not Completed (NC)	Faculty Initial with Date	Feedback Received Initial of Learner
Topic 5: Liver disease							
IM 5.15: Assist in the performance and interpret the findings of an ascitic fluid analysis							

Topic 5: Liver disease

S. No.	Name of Activity	Phase Description with Date of Completion	Attempt First (F) Repeat (R) Remedial (Re)	Rating Below Expectation (B) Meet Expectation (M)	Decision of Faculty Completed (C) Not Completed (NC)	Faculty Initial with Date	Feedback Received Initial of Learner
IM 5.14: Outline a diagnostic approach to liver disease based on hyperbilirubinemia, liver function changes and hepatitis serology							

Topic 5: Liver disease						
S. No.	Name of Activity	Phase Description with Date of Completion	Attempt First (F) Repeat (R) Remedial (Re)	Rating Below Expectation (B) Meet Expectation (M)	Decision of Faculty Completed (C) Not Completed (NC)	Faculty Initial with Date	Feedback Received Initial of Learner
IM 5.17: Enumerate the indications, precautions and counsel patients on vaccination for hepatitis						

Topic 6: HIV							
S. No.	Name of Activity	Phase Description with Date of Completion	Attempt First (F) Repeat (R) Remedial (Re)	Rating Below Expectation (B) Meet Expectation (M)	Decision of Faculty Completed (C) Not Completed (NC)	Faculty Initial with Date	Feedback Received Initial of Learner
IM 6.7: Elicit document and present a medical history that helps delineate the aetiology of the current presentation and includes risk factors for HIV, mode of infection, other sexually transmitted diseases, risks for opportunistic infections and nutritional status							

Topic 6: HIV							
S. No.	**Name of Activity**	**Phase Description with Date of Completion**	**Attempt First (F) Repeat (R) Remedial (Re)**	**Rating Below Expectation (B) Meet Expectation (M)**	**Decision of Faculty Completed (C) Not Completed (NC)**	**Faculty Initial with Date**	**Feedback Received Initial of Learner**
IM 6.8: Generate a differential diagnosis and priorities based on clinical features that suggest a specific aetiology for the presenting symptom							

S. No.	Name of Activity	Phase Description with Date of Completion	Attempt First (F) Repeat (R) Remedial (Re)	Rating Below Expectation (B) Meet Expectation (M)	Decision of Faculty Completed (C) Not Completed (NC)	Faculty Initial with Date	Feedback Received Initial of Learner
Topic 6: HIV							
IM 6.14: Perform and interpret AFB sputum							

\multicolumn{8}{c}{**Topic 6: HIV**}
S. No.	Name of Activity	Phase Description with Date of Completion	Attempt First (F) Repeat (R) Remedial (Re)	Rating Below Expectation (B) Meet Expectation (M)	Decision of Faculty Completed (C) Not Completed (NC)	Faculty Initial with Date	Feedback Received Initial of Learner
\multicolumn{8}{l}{**IM 6.15: Demonstrate in a model the correct technique to perform a lumbar puncture**}

S. No.	Name of Activity	Phase Description with Date of Completion	Attempt First (F) Repeat (R) Remedial (Re)	Rating Below Expectation (B) Meet Expectation (M)	Decision of Faculty Completed (C) Not Completed (NC)	Faculty Initial with Date	Feedback Received Initial of Learner
Topic 6: HIV							
IM 6.19: Counsel patients on prevention of HIV transmission							

		Topic 6: HIV					
S. No.	Name of Activity	Phase Description with Date of Completion	Attempt First (F) Repeat (R) Remedial (Re)	Rating Below Expectation (B) Meet Expectation (M)	Decision of Faculty Completed (C) Not Completed (NC)	Faculty Initial with Date	Feedback Received Initial of Learner
IM 6.20: Communicate diagnosis, treatment plan and subsequent follow up plan to patients							

S. No.	Name of Activity	Phase Description with Date of Completion	Attempt First (F) Repeat (R) Remedial (Re)	Rating Below Expectation (B) Meet Expectation (M)	Decision of Faculty Completed (C) Not Completed (NC)	Faculty Initial with Date	Feedback Received Initial of Learner

Topic 6: HIV

IM 6.21: Communicate with patients on the importance of medication adherence

	**Topic 6: HIV**						
S. No.	**Name of Activity**	**Phase Description with Date of Completion**	**Attempt First (F) Repeat (R) Remedial (Re)**	**Rating Below Expectation (B) Meet Expectation (M)**	**Decision of Faculty Completed (C) Not Completed (NC)**	**Faculty Initial with Date**	**Feedback Received Initial of Learner**
	**IM 6.22: Demonstrate understanding of ethical and legal issues regarding patient confidentiality and disclosure in patients with HIV**						

Topic 6: HIV						
S. No.	Name of Activity	Phase Description with Date of Completion	Attempt First (F) Repeat (R) Remedial (Re)	Rating Below Expectation (B) Meet Expectation (M)	Decision of Faculty Completed (C) Not Completed (NC)	Faculty Initial with Date	Feedback Received Initial of Learner
IM 6.23: Demonstrate a non-judgemental attitude to patients with HIV and to their lifestyles							

S. No.	Name of Activity	Phase Description with Date of Completion	Attempt First (F) Repeat (R) Remedial (Re)	Rating Below Expectation (B) Meet Expectation (M)	Decision of Faculty Completed (C) Not Completed (NC)	Faculty Initial with Date	Feedback Received Initial of Learner
colspan over Topic 7: Rheumatologic Diseases							

Topic 7: Rheumatologic Diseases

IM 7.11: Elicit document and present a medical history that will differentiate the aetiologies of disease

Topic 7: Rheumatologic Diseases							
S. No.	Name of Activity	Phase Description with Date of Completion	Attempt First (F) Repeat (R) Remedial (Re)	Rating Below Expectation (B) Meet Expectation (M)	Decision of Faculty Completed (C) Not Completed (NC)	Faculty Initial with Date	Feedback Received Initial of Learner
IM 7.12: Perform a systematic examination of y all joints, muscle and skin that will establish the diagnosis and severity of disease							

Topic 7: Rheumatologic Diseases						
S. No.	Name of Activity	Phase Description with Date of Completion	Attempt First (F) Repeat (R) Remedial (Re)	Rating Below Expectation (B) Meet Expectation (M)	Decision of Faculty Completed (C) Not Completed (NC)	Faculty Initial with Date	Feedback Received Initial of Learner
IM 7.15: Enumerate the indications for and interpret the results of : CBC, anti- CCP, RA, ANA, DNA and other tests of autoimmunity							

	Topic 7: Rheumatologic Diseases						
S. No.	Name of Activity	Phase Description with Date of Completion	Attempt First (F) Repeat (R) Remedial (Re)	Rating Below Expectation (B) Meet Expectation (M)	Decision of Faculty Completed (C) Not Completed (NC)	Faculty Initial with Date	Feedback Received Initial of Learner
IM 7.17: Enumerate the indications and interpret plain radiographs of joints							

S. No.	Name of Activity	Phase Description with Date of Completion	Attempt First (F) Repeat (R) Remedial (Re)	Rating Below Expectation (B) Meet Expectation (M)	Decision of Faculty Completed (C) Not Completed (NC)	Faculty Initial with Date	Feedback Received Initial of Learner
Topic 7: Rheumatologic Diseases							
IM 7.18: Communicate diagnosis, treatment plan and subsequent follow up plan to patients							

S. No.	Name of Activity	Phase Description with Date of Completion	Attempt First (F) Repeat (R) Remedial (Re)	Rating Below Expectation (B) Meet Expectation (M)	Decision of Faculty Completed (C) Not Completed (NC)	Faculty Initial with Date	Feedback Received Initial of Learner

Topic 7: Rheumatologic Diseases

IM 7.20: Select, prescribe and communicate appropriate medications for relief of joint pain

S. No.	Name of Activity	Phase Description with Date of Completion	Attempt First (F) Repeat (R) Remedial (Re)	Rating Below Expectation (B) Meet Expectation (M)	Decision of Faculty Completed (C) Not Completed (NC)	Faculty Initial with Date	Feedback Received Initial of Learner
Topic 7: Rheumatologic Diseases							
IM 7.21: Select, prescribe and communicate preventive therapy for crystalline arthropathies							

S. No.	Name of Activity	Phase Description with Date of Completion	Attempt First (F) Repeat (R) Remedial (Re)	Rating Below Expectation (B) Meet Expectation (M)	Decision of Faculty Completed (C) Not Completed (NC)	Faculty Initial with Date	Feedback Received Initial of Learner
Topic 7: Rheumatologic Diseases							
IM 7.22: Select, prescribe and communicate treatment option for systemic rheumatologic conditions							

Topic 7: Rheumatologic Diseases							
S. No.	Name of Activity	Phase Description with Date of Completion	Attempt First (F) Repeat (R) Remedial (Re)	Rating Below Expectation (B) Meet Expectation (M)	Decision of Faculty Completed (C) Not Completed (NC)	Faculty Initial with Date	Feedback Received Initial of Learner
IM 7.24: Communicate and incorporate patient preferences in the choice of therapy							

S. No.	Name of Activity	Phase Description with Date of Completion	Attempt First (F) Repeat (R) Remedial (Re)	Rating Below Expectation (B) Meet Expectation (M)	Decision of Faculty Completed (C) Not Completed (NC)	Faculty Initial with Date	Feedback Received Initial of Learner
Topic 7: Rheumatologic Diseases							
IM 7.25: Develop and communicate appropriate follow up and monitoring plans for patients with rheumatologic conditions							

Topic 7: Rheumatologic Diseases							
S. No.	Name of Activity	Phase Description with Date of Completion	Attempt First (F) Repeat (R) Remedial (Re)	Rating Below Expectation (B) Meet Expectation (M)	Decision of Faculty Completed (C) Not Completed (NC)	Faculty Initial with Date	Feedback Received Initial of Learner
IM 7.26: Demonstrate an understanding of the impact of rheumatologic conditions on quality of life, wellbeing, work and family							

Topic 8: Hypertension

S. No.	Name of Activity	Phase Description with Date of Completion	Attempt First (F) Repeat (R) Remedial (Re)	Rating Below Expectation (B) Meet Expectation (M)	Decision of Faculty Completed (C) Not Completed (NC)	Faculty Initial with Date	Feedback Received Initial of Learner
IM 8.9: Elicit document and present a medical history that includes: duration and levels, symptoms, comorbidities, lifestyle, risk factors, family history, psychosocial and environmental factors, dietary assessment, previous and concomitant therapy							

S. No.	Name of Activity	Phase Description with Date of Completion	Attempt First (F) Repeat (R) Remedial (Re)	Rating Below Expectation (B) Meet Expectation (M)	Decision of Faculty Completed (C) Not Completed (NC)	Faculty Initial with Date	Feedback Received Initial of Learner
	**Topic 8: Hypertension**
	**IM 8.10: Perform a systematic examination that includes : an accurate measurement of blood pressure, fundus examination, examination of vasculature and heart**

S. No.	Name of Activity	Phase Description with Date of Completion	Attempt First (F) Repeat (R) Remedial (Re)	Rating Below Expectation (B) Meet Expectation (M)	Decision of Faculty Completed (C) Not Completed (NC)	Faculty Initial with Date	Feedback Received Initial of Learner
Topic 8: Hypertension							
IM 8.11: Generate a differential diagnosis and priorities based on clinical features that suggest a specific aetiology							

S. No.	Name of Activity	Phase Description with Date of Completion	Attempt First (F) Repeat (R) Remedial (Re)	Rating Below Expectation (B) Meet Expectation (M)	Decision of Faculty Completed (C) Not Completed (NC)	Faculty Initial with Date	Feedback Received Initial of Learner
Topic 8: Hypertension							
IM 8.15: Recognize, priorities and manage hypertensive emergencies							

	Topic 8: Hypertension						
S. No.	Name of Activity	Phase Description with Date of Completion	Attempt First (F) Repeat (R) Remedial (Re)	Rating Below Expectation (B) Meet Expectation (M)	Decision of Faculty Completed (C) Not Completed (NC)	Faculty Initial with Date	Feedback Received Initial of Learner
IM 8.16: Develop and communicate to the patient lifestyle modification including weight reduction, moderation of alcohol intake, physical activity and sodium intake							

Topic 8: Hypertension							
S. No.	Name of Activity	Phase Description with Date of Completion	Attempt First (F) Repeat (R) Remedial (Re)	Rating Below Expectation (B) Meet Expectation (M)	Decision of Faculty Completed (C) Not Completed (NC)	Faculty Initial with Date	Feedback Received Initial of Learner
IM 8.18: Incorporate patient preferences in the management of HTN							

S. No.	Name of Activity	Phase Description with Date of Completion	Attempt First (F) Repeat (R) Remedial (Re)	Rating Below Expectation (B) Meet Expectation (M)	Decision of Faculty Completed (C) Not Completed (NC)	Faculty Initial with Date	Feedback Received Initial of Learner
	**Topic 8: Hypertension**
	**IM 8.19**: Demonstrate understanding of the impact of Hypertension on quality of life, wellbeing, work and family

Topic 9: Anemia							
S. No.	Name of Activity	Phase Description with Date of Completion	Attempt First (F) Repeat (R) Remedial (Re)	Rating Below Expectation (B) Meet Expectation (M)	Decision of Faculty Completed (C) Not Completed (NC)	Faculty Initial with Date	Feedback Received Initial of Learner
IM 9.3: Elicit document and present a medical history that includes symptoms, risk factors including GI bleeding, prior history, medications, menstrual history, and family history							

Topic 9: Anemia

S. No.	Name of Activity	Phase Description with Date of Completion	Attempt First (F) Repeat (R) Remedial (Re)	Rating Below Expectation (B) Meet Expectation (M)	Decision of Faculty Completed (C) Not Completed (NC)	Faculty Initial with Date	Feedback Received Initial of Learner
IM 9.4: Perform a systematic examination that includes : general examination for pallor, oral examination, DOAP session of hyper dynamic circulation, lymph node and splenic examination							

Topic 9: Anemia							
S. No.	**Name of Activity**	**Phase Description with Date of Completion**	**Attempt First (F) Repeat (R) Remedial (Re)**	**Rating Below Expectation (B) Meet Expectation (M)**	**Decision of Faculty Completed (C) Not Completed (NC)**	**Faculty Initial with Date**	**Feedback Received Initial of Learner**
IM 9.5: Generate a differential diagnosis and priorities based on clinical features that suggest a specific aetiology							

S. No.	Name of Activity	Phase Description with Date of Completion	Attempt First (F) Repeat (R) Remedial (Re)	Rating Below Expectation (B) Meet Expectation (M)	Decision of Faculty Completed (C) Not Completed (NC)	Faculty Initial with Date	Feedback Received Initial of Learner
Topic 9: Anemia							
IM 9.6: Describe the appropriate diagnostic work up based on the presumed aetiology							

Topic 9: Anemia							
S. No.	Name of Activity	Phase Description with Date of Completion	Attempt First (F) Repeat (R) Remedial (Re)	Rating Below Expectation (B) Meet Expectation (M)	Decision of Faculty Completed (C) Not Completed (NC)	Faculty Initial with Date	Feedback Received Initial of Learner
IM 9.9: Order and interpret tests for anemia including hemogram, red cell indices, reticulocyte count, iron studies, B12 and folate							

Topic 9: Anemia							
S. No.	Name of Activity	Phase Description with Date of Completion	Attempt First (F) Repeat (R) Remedial (Re)	Rating Below Expectation (B) Meet Expectation (M)	Decision of Faculty Completed (C) Not Completed (NC)	Faculty Initial with Date	Feedback Received Initial of Learner
IM 9.10: Describe, perform and interpret a peripheral smear and stool occult blood							

\n S. No.	Name of Activity	Phase Description with Date of Completion	Attempt First (F) Repeat (R) Remedial (Re)	Rating Below Expectation (B) Meet Expectation (M)	Decision of Faculty Completed (C) Not Completed (NC)	Faculty Initial with Date	Feedback Received\n\nInitial of Learner
IM 9.13: Prescribe replacement therapy with iron, B12, folate							

Topic 9: Anemia

S. No.	Name of Activity	Phase Description with Date of Completion	Attempt First (F) Repeat (R) Remedial (Re)	Rating Below Expectation (B) Meet Expectation (M)	Decision of Faculty Completed (C) Not Completed (NC)	Faculty Initial with Date	Feedback Received Initial of Learner
Topic 9: Anemia							
IM 9.15: Communicate the diagnosis and the treatment appropriately to patients							

S. No.	Name of Activity	Phase Description with Date of Completion	Attempt First (F) Repeat (R) Remedial (Re)	Rating Below Expectation (B) Meet Expectation (M)	Decision of Faculty Completed (C) Not Completed (NC)	Faculty Initial with Date	Feedback Received Initial of Learner
Topic 9: Anemia							
IM 9.16: Incorporate patient preferences in the management of anemia							

				Topic 9: Anemia			
S. No.	Name of Activity	Phase Description with Date of Completion	Attempt First (F) Repeat (R) Remedial (Re)	Rating Below Expectation (B) Meet Expectation (M)	Decision of Faculty Completed (C) Not Completed (NC)	Faculty Initial with Date	Feedback Received Initial of Learner
IM 9.19: Assist in a blood transfusion							

S. No.	Name of Activity	Phase Description with Date of Completion	Attempt First (F) Repeat (R) Remedial (Re)	Rating Below Expectation (B) Meet Expectation (M)	Decision of Faculty Completed (C) Not Completed (NC)	Faculty Initial with Date	Feedback Received Initial of Learner
IM 9.20: Communicate and counsel patients with methods to prevent nutritional anemia							

Topic 9: Anemia

S. No.	Name of Activity	Phase Description with Date of Completion	Attempt First (F) Repeat (R) Remedial (Re)	Rating Below Expectation (B) Meet Expectation (M)	Decision of Faculty Completed (C) Not Completed (NC)	Faculty Initial with Date	Feedback Received Initial of Learner
IM 10.12: Elicit document and present a medical history that will differentiate the aetiologies of disease, distinguish acute and chronic disease, identify predisposing conditions, nephrotoxic drugs and systemic causes

Topic 10: Acute Kidney Injury and Chronic renal failure

Topic 10: Acute Kidney Injury and Chronic renal failure							
S. No.	**Name of Activity**	**Phase Description with Date of Completion**	**Attempt First (F) Repeat (R) Remedial (Re)**	**Rating Below Expectation (B) Meet Expectation (M)**	**Decision of Faculty Completed (C) Not Completed (NC)**	**Faculty Initial with Date**	**Feedback Received Initial of Learner**
IM 10.13: Perform a systematic examination that establishes the diagnosis and severity including determination of volume status, presence of edema and heart failure, features of uraemia and associated systemic disease							

S. No.	Name of Activity	Phase Description with Date of Completion	Attempt First (F) Repeat (R) Remedial (Re)	Rating Below Expectation (B) Meet Expectation (M)	Decision of Faculty Completed (C) Not Completed (NC)	Faculty Initial with Date	Feedback Received Initial of Learner
Topic 10: Acute Kidney Injury and Chronic renal failure							
IM 10.15: Describe the appropriate diagnostic work up based on the presumed aetiology							

Topic 10: Acute Kidney Injury and Chronic renal failure

S. No.	Name of Activity	Phase Description with Date of Completion	Attempt First (F) Repeat (R) Remedial (Re)	Rating Below Expectation (B) Meet Expectation (M)	Decision of Faculty Completed (C) Not Completed (NC)	Faculty Initial with Date	Feedback Received Initial of Learner
IM10.14: Generate a differential diagnosis and prioritise based on clinical features that suggest a specific aetiology							

S. No.	Name of Activity	Phase Description with Date of Completion	Attempt First (F) Repeat (R) Remedial (Re)	Rating Below Expectation (B) Meet Expectation (M)	Decision of Faculty Completed (C) Not Completed (NC)	Faculty Initial with Date	Feedback Received Initial of Learner
colspan with Topic 10 heading above							

Topic 10: Acute Kidney Injury and Chronic renal failure

S. No.	Name of Activity	Phase Description with Date of Completion	Attempt First (F) Repeat (R) Remedial (Re)	Rating Below Expectation (B) Meet Expectation (M)	Decision of Faculty Completed (C) Not Completed (NC)	Faculty Initial with Date	Feedback Received Initial of Learner
IM 10.17: Describe and calculate indices of renal function based on available laboratories including FENa (Fractional Excretion of Sodium) and CrCl (Creatinine Clearance)							

S. No.	Name of Activity	Phase Description with Date of Completion	Attempt First (F) Repeat (R) Remedial (Re)	Rating Below Expectation (B) Meet Expectation (M)	Decision of Faculty Completed (C) Not Completed (NC)	Faculty Initial with Date	Feedback Received Initial of Learner
Topic 10: Acute Kidney Injury and Chronic renal failure							
IM 10.18: Identify the ECG findings in hyperkalemia							

S. No.	Name of Activity	Phase Description with Date of Completion	Attempt First (F) Repeat (R) Remedial (Re)	Rating Below Expectation (B) Meet Expectation (M)	Decision of Faculty Completed (C) Not Completed (NC)	Faculty Initial with Date	Feedback Received Initial of Learner
	**Topic 10: Acute Kidney Injury and Chronic renal failure**
	**IM 10.20: Describe and discuss the indications to perform arterial blood gas analysis: interpret the data**

S. No.	Name of Activity	Phase Description with Date of Completion	Attempt First (F) Repeat (R) Remedial (Re)	Rating Below Expectation (B) Meet Expectation (M)	Decision of Faculty Completed (C) Not Completed (NC)	Faculty Initial with Date	Feedback Received Initial of Learner
Topic 10: Acute Kidney Injury and Chronic renal failure							
IM 10.16: Enumerate the indications for and interpret the results of : renal function tests, calcium, phosphorus, PTH, urine electrolytes, osmolality, Anion gap							

Topic 10: Acute Kidney Injury and Chronic renal failure

S. No.	Name of Activity	Phase Description with Date of Completion	Attempt First (F) Repeat (R) Remedial (Re)	Rating Below Expectation (B) Meet Expectation (M)	Decision of Faculty Completed (C) Not Completed (NC)	Faculty Initial with Date	Feedback Received Initial of Learner
IM 10.21: Describe and discuss the indications for and insert a peripheral intravenous catheter							

Topic 10: Acute Kidney Injury and Chronic renal failure

S. No.	Name of Activity	Phase Description with Date of Completion	Attempt First (F) Repeat (R) Remedial (Re)	Rating Below Expectation (B) Meet Expectation (M)	Decision of Faculty Completed (C) Not Completed (NC)	Faculty Initial with Date	Feedback Received Initial of Learner
IM 10.22: Describe and discuss the indications, demonstrate in a model and assist in the insertion of a central venous or a dialysis catheter							

S. No.	Name of Activity	Phase Description with Date of Completion	Attempt First (F) Repeat (R) Remedial (Re)	Rating Below Expectation (B) Meet Expectation (M)	Decision of Faculty Completed (C) Not Completed (NC)	Faculty Initial with Date	Feedback Received Initial of Learner
Topic 10: Acute Kidney Injury and Chronic renal failure							
IM 10.23: Communicate diagnosis treatment plan and subsequent follow up plan to patients							

S. No.	Name of Activity	Phase Description with Date of Completion	Attempt First (F) Repeat (R) Remedial (Re)	Rating Below Expectation (B) Meet Expectation (M)	Decision of Faculty Completed (C) Not Completed (NC)	Faculty Initial with Date	Feedback Received Initial of Learner
Topic 10: Acute Kidney Injury and Chronic renal failure							
IM 10.24: Counsel patients on a renal diet							

S. No.	Name of Activity	Phase Description with Date of Completion	Attempt First (F) Repeat (R) Remedial (Re)	Rating Below Expectation (B) Meet Expectation (M)	Decision of Faculty Completed (C) Not Completed (NC)	Faculty Initial with Date	Feedback Received Initial of Learner
Topic 11: Diabetes Mellitus							
IM 11.7: Elicit document and present a medical history that will differentiate the aetiologies of diabetes including risk factors, precipitating factors, lifestyle, nutritional history, family history, medication history, co-morbidities and target organ disease							

Topic 11: Diabetes Mellitus							
S. No.	**Name of Activity**	**Phase Description with Date of Completion**	**Attempt First (F) Repeat (R) Remedial (Re)**	**Rating Below Expectation (B) Meet Expectation (M)**	**Decision of Faculty Completed (C) Not Completed (NC)**	**Faculty Initial with Date**	**Feedback Received** **Initial of Learner**
IM 11.8: Perform a systematic examination that establishes the diagnosis and severity that includes skin, peripheral pulses, blood pressure measurement, fundus examination, detailed examination of the foot (pulses, nervous and deformities and injuries)							

Topic 11: Diabetes Mellitus							
S. No.	Name of Activity	Phase Description with Date of Completion	Attempt First (F) Repeat (R) Remedial (Re)	Rating Below Expectation (B) Meet Expectation (M)	Decision of Faculty Completed (C) Not Completed (NC)	Faculty Initial with Date	Feedback Received Initial of Learner
IM 11.11: Order and interpret laboratory tests to diagnose diabetes and its complications including: glucoses, glucose tolerance test, glycosylated hemoglobin, urinary micro albumin, ECG, electrolytes, ABG, ketones, renal function tests and lipid profile							

Topic 11: Diabetes Mellitus							
S. No.	Name of Activity	Phase Description with Date of Completion	Attempt First (F) Repeat (R) Remedial (Re)	Rating Below Expectation (B) Meet Expectation (M)	Decision of Faculty Completed (C) Not Completed (NC)	Faculty Initial with Date	Feedback Received Initial of Learner
IM 11.19: Demonstrate and counsel patients on the correct technique to administer insulin							

S. No.	Name of Activity	Phase Description with Date of Completion	Attempt First (F) Repeat (R) Remedial (Re)	Rating Below Expectation (B) Meet Expectation (M)	Decision of Faculty Completed (C) Not Completed (NC)	Faculty Initial with Date	Feedback Received Initial of Learner
IM 11.20: Demonstrate to and counsel patients correct technique on the of self-monitoring of blood glucoses							

S. No.	Name of Activity	Phase Description with Date of Completion	Attempt First (F) Repeat (R) Remedial (Re)	Rating Below Expectation (B) Meet Expectation (M)	Decision of Faculty Completed (C) Not Completed (NC)	Faculty Initial with Date	Feedback Received Initial of Learner
Topic 11: Diabetes Mellitus							
IM 11.21: Recognise the importance of patient preference while selecting therapy for diabetes							

S. No.	Name of Activity	Phase Description with Date of Completion	Attempt First (F) Repeat (R) Remedial (Re)	Rating Below Expectation (B) Meet Expectation (M)	Decision of Faculty Completed (C) Not Completed (NC)	Faculty Initial with Date	Feedback Received Initial of Learner
Topic 12: Thyroid disorders							
IM 12.5: Elicit document and present an appropriate history that will establish the diagnosis cause of thyroid dysfunction and its severity							

Topic 12: Thyroid disorders

S. No.	Name of Activity	Phase Description with Date of Completion	Attempt First (F) Repeat (R) Remedial (Re)	Rating Below Expectation (B) Meet Expectation (M)	Decision of Faculty Completed (C) Not Completed (NC)	Faculty Initial with Date	Feedback Received Initial of Learner
IM 12.6: Perform and demonstrate a systematic examination based on the history that will help establish the diagnosis and severity including systemic signs of thyrotoxicosis and hypothyroidism, palpation of the pulse for rate & rhythm abnormalities, neck palpation of the thyroid and lymph nodes and cardiovascular findings							

S. No.	Name of Activity	Phase Description with Date of Completion	Attempt First (F) Repeat (R) Remedial (Re)	Rating Below Expectation (B) Meet Expectation (M)	Decision of Faculty Completed (C) Not Completed (NC)	Faculty Initial with Date	Feedback Received Initial of Learner
Topic 12: Thyroid disorders							
IM 12.7: Demonstrate the correct technique to palpate the thyroid							

Topic 12: Thyroid disorders							
S. No.	Name of Activity	Phase Description with Date of Completion	Attempt First (F) Repeat (R) Remedial (Re)	Rating Below Expectation (B) Meet Expectation (M)	Decision of Faculty Completed (C) Not Completed (NC)	Faculty Initial with Date	Feedback Received Initial of Learner
IM 12.8: Generate a differential diagnosis based on the clinical presentation and prioritise it based on the most likely diagnosis							

Topic 12: Thyroid disorders

S. No.	Name of Activity	Phase Description with Date of Completion	Attempt First (F) Repeat (R) Remedial (Re)	Rating Below Expectation (B) Meet Expectation (M)	Decision of Faculty Completed (C) Not Completed (NC)	Faculty Initial with Date	Feedback Received Initial of Learner
IM 12.9: Order and interpret diagnostic testing based on the clinical diagnosis including CBC, thyroid function tests and ECG and radio iodine uptake and scan							

Topic 12: Thyroid disorders

S. No.	Name of Activity	Phase Description with Date of Completion	Attempt First (F) Repeat (R) Remedial (Re)	Rating Below Expectation (B) Meet Expectation (M)	Decision of Faculty Completed (C) Not Completed (NC)	Faculty Initial with Date	Feedback Received Initial of Learner
IM 12.10: Identify atrial fibrillation, pericardial effusion and bradycardia on ECG							

Topic 12: Thyroid disorders

S. No.	Name of Activity	Phase Description with Date of Completion	Attempt First (F) Repeat (R) Remedial (Re)	Rating Below Expectation (B) Meet Expectation (M)	Decision of Faculty Completed (C) Not Completed (NC)	Faculty Initial with Date	Feedback Received Initial of Learner
IM 12.11: Interpret thyroid function tests in hypo and hyperthyroidism							

S. No.	Name of Activity	Phase Description with Date of Completion	Attempt First (F) Repeat (R) Remedial (Re)	Rating Below Expectation (B) Meet Expectation (M)	Decision of Faculty Completed (C) Not Completed (NC)	Faculty Initial with Date	Feedback Received Initial of Learner
IM 12.14: Write and communicate to the patient appropriately a prescription for thyroxine based on age, sex, and clinical and biochemical status							

Topic 12: Thyroid disorders

S. No.	Name of Activity	Phase Description with Date of Completion	Attempt First (F) Repeat (R) Remedial (Re)	Rating Below Expectation (B) Meet Expectation (M)	Decision of Faculty Completed (C) Not Completed (NC)	Faculty Initial with Date	Feedback Received Initial of Learner
Topic 13: Malignancies							
IM 13.8: Perform and demonstrate a physical examination that includes an appropriate general and local examination that excludes the diagnosis, extent spread and complications of cancer							

Topic 14: Obesity

S. No.	Name of Activity	Phase Description with Date of Completion	Attempt First (F) Repeat (R) Remedial (Re)	Rating Below Expectation (B) Meet Expectation (M)	Decision of Faculty Completed (C) Not Completed (NC)	Faculty Initial with Date	Feedback Received Initial of Learner
IM 14.6: Elicit and document and present an appropriate history that includes the natural history, dietary history, modifiable risk factors, family history clues for secondary causes and motivation to lose weight							

S. No.	Name of Activity	Phase Description with Date of Completion	Attempt First (F) Repeat (R) Remedial (Re)	Rating Below Expectation (B) Meet Expectation (M)	Decision of Faculty Completed (C) Not Completed (NC)	Faculty Initial with Date	Feedback Received Initial of Learner

Topic 14: Obesity

IM 14.7: Perform, document and demonstrate a physical examination based on the history that includes general examination, measurement of abdominal obesity, signs of secondary causes and comorbidities

S. No.	Name of Activity	Phase Description with Date of Completion	Attempt First (F) Repeat (R) Remedial (Re)	Rating Below Expectation (B) Meet Expectation (M)	Decision of Faculty Completed (C) Not Completed (NC)	Faculty Initial with Date	Feedback Received Initial of Learner
	**Topic 14: Obesity**
	IM 14.8: Generate a differential diagnosis based on the presenting symptoms and clinical features and priorities based on the most likely diagnosis

				Topic 14: Obesity			
S. No.	Name of Activity	Phase Description with Date of Completion	Attempt First (F) Repeat (R) Remedial (Re)	Rating Below Expectation (B) Meet Expectation (M)	Decision of Faculty Completed (C) Not Completed (NC)	Faculty Initial with Date	Feedback Received Initial of Learner
IM 14.9: Order and interpret diagnostic tests based on the clinical diagnosis including blood glucose, lipids, thyroid function tests etc.							

Topic 14: Obesity							
S. No.	Name of Activity	Phase Description with Date of Completion	Attempt First (F) Repeat (R) Remedial (Re)	Rating Below Expectation (B) Meet Expectation (M)	Decision of Faculty Completed (C) Not Completed (NC)	Faculty Initial with Date	Feedback Received Initial of Learner
IM 14.11: Communicate and counsel patient on behavioral, dietary and lifestyle modifications							

Topic 14: Obesity							
S. No.	Name of Activity	Phase Description with Date of Completion	Attempt First (F) Repeat (R) Remedial (Re)	Rating Below Expectation (B) Meet Expectation (M)	Decision of Faculty Completed (C) Not Completed (NC)	Faculty Initial with Date	Feedback Received Initial of Learner
IM 14.12: Demonstrate an understanding of patient's inability to adhere to lifestyle instructions and counsel them in a non - judgmental way							

Topic 15: Gastro-intestinal Bleeding						
S. No.	Name of Activity	Phase Description with Date of Completion	Attempt First (F) Repeat (R) Remedial (Re)	Rating Below Expectation (B) Meet Expectation (M)	Decision of Faculty Completed (C) Not Completed (NC)	Faculty Initial with Date	Feedback Received Initial of Learner
IM 15.2: Enumerate, describe and discuss the evaluation and steps involved in stabilizing a patient who presents with acute volume loss and GI bleed							

Topic 15: Gastro-intestinal Bleeding						
S. No.	Name of Activity	Phase Description with Date of Completion	Attempt First (F) Repeat (R) Remedial (Re)	Rating Below Expectation (B) Meet Expectation (M)	Decision of Faculty Completed (C) Not Completed (NC)	Faculty Initial with Date	Feedback Received Initial of Learner
IM 15.4: Elicit and document and present an appropriate history that identifies the route of bleeding, quantity, grade, volume loss, duration, etiology, comorbid illnesses and risk factors							

Topic 15: Gastro-intestinal Bleeding							
S. No.	Name of Activity	Phase Description with Date of Completion	Attempt First (F) Repeat (R) Remedial (Re)	Rating Below Expectation (B) Meet Expectation (M)	Decision of Faculty Completed (C) Not Completed (NC)	Faculty Initial with Date	Feedback Received Initial of Learner
IM 15.5: Perform, demonstrate and document a physical examination based on the history that includes general examination, volume assessment and appropriate abdominal examination							

Topic 15: Gastro-intestinal Bleeding							
S. No.	Name of Activity	Phase Description with Date of Completion	Attempt First (F) Repeat (R) Remedial (Re)	Rating Below Expectation (B) Meet Expectation (M)	Decision of Faculty Completed (C) Not Completed (NC)	Faculty Initial with Date	Feedback Received Initial of Learner
IM 15.7: Demonstrate the correct technique to perform q p an anal and rectal							

Topic 15: Gastro-intestinal Bleeding

S. No.	Name of Activity	Phase Description with Date of Completion	Attempt First (F) Repeat (R) Remedial (Re)	Rating Below Expectation (B) Meet Expectation (M)	Decision of Faculty Completed (C) Not Completed (NC)	Faculty Initial with Date	Feedback Received Initial of Learner
IM 15.8: Generate a differential diagnosis based on the presenting symptoms and clinical features and priorities based on the most likely diagnosis							

S. No.	Name of Activity	Phase Description with Date of Completion	Attempt First (F) Repeat (R) Remedial (Re)	Rating Below Expectation (B) Meet Expectation (M)	Decision of Faculty Completed (C) Not Completed (NC)	Faculty Initial with Date	Feedback Received Initial of Learner

Topic 15: Gastro-intestinal Bleeding

IM 15.9: Choose and interpret diagnostic tests based on the clinical diagnosis including complete blood count, PT and PTT, stool examination, occult blood, liver function tests, H.pylori test.

		Topic 15: Gastro-intestinal Bleeding					
S. No.	Name of Activity	Phase Description with Date of Completion	Attempt First (F) Repeat (R) Remedial (Re)	Rating Below Expectation (B) Meet Expectation (M)	Decision of Faculty Completed (C) Not Completed (NC)	Faculty Initial with Date	Feedback Received Initial of Learner
IM 15.13: Observe cross matching and blood / blood component transfusion							

S. No.	Name of Activity	Phase Description with Date of Completion	Attempt First (F) Repeat (R) Remedial (Re)	Rating Below Expectation (B) Meet Expectation (M)	Decision of Faculty Completed (C) Not Completed (NC)	Faculty Initial with Date	Feedback Received Initial of Learner
Topic 15: Gastro-intestinal Bleeding							
IM 15.18: Counsel the family and patient in an empathetic non-judgmental manner on the diagnosis and therapeutic options							

| \multicolumn{8}{c}{**Topic 16: Diarrheal disorder**} |

S. No.	Name of Activity	Phase Description with Date of Completion	Attempt First (F) Repeat (R) Remedial (Re)	Rating Below Expectation (B) Meet Expectation (M)	Decision of Faculty Completed (C) Not Completed (NC)	Faculty Initial with Date	Feedback Received Initial of Learner
\multicolumn{8}{l}{**IM 16.4: Elicit and document and present an appropriate history that includes the natural history, dietary history, travel , sexual history and other concomitant illnesses**}

Topic 16: Diarrheal disorder							
S. No.	Name of Activity	Phase Description with Date of Completion	Attempt First (F) Repeat (R) Remedial (Re)	Rating Below Expectation (B) Meet Expectation (M)	Decision of Faculty Completed (C) Not Completed (NC)	Faculty Initial with Date	Feedback Received Initial of Learner
IM 16.5: Perform, document and demonstrate a physical examination based on the history that includes general examination, including an appropriate abdominal examination							

Topic 16: Diarrheal disorder							
S. No.	**Name of Activity**	**Phase Description with Date of Completion**	**Attempt First (F) Repeat (R) Remedial (Re)**	**Rating Below Expectation (B) Meet Expectation (M)**	**Decision of Faculty Completed (C) Not Completed (NC)**	**Faculty Initial with Date**	**Feedback Received Initial of Learner**
IM 16.7: Generate a differential diagnosis based on the presenting symptoms and clinical features and priorities based on the most likely diagnosis							

S. No.	Name of Activity	Phase Description with Date of Completion	Attempt First (F) Repeat (R) Remedial (Re)	Rating Below Expectation (B) Meet Expectation (M)	Decision of Faculty Completed (C) Not Completed (NC)	Faculty Initial with Date	Feedback Received Initial of Learner
Topic 16: Diarrheal disorder							
IM 16.8: Choose and interpret diagnostic tests based on the clinical diagnosis including complete blood count, and stool examination							

			Topic 16: Diarrheal disorder				
S. No.	Name of Activity	Phase Description with Date of Completion	Attempt First (F) Repeat (R) Remedial (Re)	Rating Below Expectation (B) Meet Expectation (M)	Decision of Faculty Completed (C) Not Completed (NC)	Faculty Initial with Date	Feedback Received Initial of Learner
IM 16.9: Identify common parasitic causes of diarrhea under the microscope in a stool specimen							

Topic 16: Diarrheal disorder						
S. No.	Name of Activity	Phase Description with Date of Completion	Attempt First (F) Repeat (R) Remedial (Re)	Rating Below Expectation (B) Meet Expectation (M)	Decision of Faculty Completed (C) Not Completed (NC)	Faculty Initial with Date	Feedback Received Initial of Learner
IM 16.10: Identify vibrio cholera in a hanging drop specimen							

Topic 16: Diarrheal disorder						
S. No.	Name of Activity	Phase Description with Date of Completion	Attempt First (F) Repeat (R) Remedial (Re)	Rating Below Expectation (B) Meet Expectation (M)	Decision of Faculty Completed (C) Not Completed (NC)	Faculty Initial with Date	Feedback Received Initial of Learner
IM 16.15: Distinguish based on the clinical presentation Crohn's disease from Ulcerative Colitis							

Topic 17: Headache

S. No.	Name of Activity	Phase Description with Date of Completion	Attempt First (F) Repeat (R) Remedial (Re)	Rating Below Expectation (B) Meet Expectation (M)	Decision of Faculty Completed (C) Not Completed (NC)	Faculty Initial with Date	Feedback Received Initial of Learner
IM 17.2: Elicit and document and present an appropriate history including aura, precipitating aggravating and relieving factors, associated symptoms that help identify the cause of headaches							

S. No.	Name of Activity	Phase Description with Date of Completion	Attempt First (F) Repeat (R) Remedial (Re)	Rating Below Expectation (B) Meet Expectation (M)	Decision of Faculty Completed (C) Not Completed (NC)	Faculty Initial with Date	Feedback Received Initial of Learner
Topic 17: Headache							
IM 17.4: Perform and demonstrate a general neurologic examination and a focused examination for signs of intracranial tension including neck signs of meningitis							

Topic 17: Headache							
S. No.	**Name of Activity**	**Phase Description with Date of Completion**	**Attempt First (F) Repeat (R) Remedial (Re)**	**Rating Below Expectation (B) Meet Expectation (M)**	**Decision of Faculty Completed (C) Not Completed (NC)**	**Faculty Initial with Date**	**Feedback Received Initial of Learner**
IM 17.5: Generate document and present a differential diagnosis based on the clinical feature and priorities the diagnosis based on the presentation							

S. No.	Name of Activity	Phase Description with Date of Completion	Attempt First (F) Repeat (R) Remedial (Re)	Rating Below Expectation (B) Meet Expectation (M)	Decision of Faculty Completed (C) Not Completed (NC)	Faculty Initial with Date	Feedback Received Initial of Learner
Topic 17: Headache							
IM 17.6: Choose and interpret diagnostic testing based on the clinical diagnosis including imaging							

				Topic 17: Headache			
S. No.	Name of Activity	Phase Description with Date of Completion	Attempt First (F) Repeat (R) Remedial (Re)	Rating Below Expectation (B) Meet Expectation (M)	Decision of Faculty Completed (C) Not Completed (NC)	Faculty Initial with Date	Feedback Received Initial of Learner
IM 17.8: Demonstrate in a mannequin or equivalent the correct technique for performing a lumbar puncture							

S. No.	Name of Activity	Phase Description with Date of Completion	Attempt First (F) Repeat (R) Remedial (Re)	Rating Below Expectation (B) Meet Expectation (M)	Decision of Faculty Completed (C) Not Completed (NC)	Faculty Initial with Date	Feedback Received Initial of Learner
Topic 17: Headache							
IM 17.9: Interpret the CSF findings when presented with various parameters of CSF fluid analysis							

Topic 17: Headache							
S. No.	Name of Activity	Phase Description with Date of Completion	Attempt First (F) Repeat (R) Remedial (Re)	Rating Below Expectation (B) Meet Expectation (M)	Decision of Faculty Completed (C) Not Completed (NC)	Faculty Initial with Date	Feedback Received Initial of Learner
IM 17.14: Counsel patients with migraine and tension headache on lifestyle changes and need for prophylactic therapy							

Topic 18: Cerebrovascular accident						
S. No.	Name of Activity	Phase Description with Date of Completion	Attempt First (F) Repeat (R) Remedial (Re)	Rating Below Expectation (B) Meet Expectation (M)	Decision of Faculty Completed (C) Not Completed (NC)	Faculty Initial with Date	Feedback Received Initial of Learner
IM 18.3: Elicit and document and present an appropriate history including onset, progression, precipitating and aggravating relieving factors, associated symptoms that help identify the cause of the cerebrovascular accident							

Topic 18: Cerebrovascular accident

S. No.	Name of Activity	Phase Description with Date of Completion	Attempt First (F) Repeat (R) Remedial (Re)	Rating Below Expectation (B) Meet Expectation (M)	Decision of Faculty Completed (C) Not Completed (NC)	Faculty Initial with Date	Feedback Received Initial of Learner
IM 18.5: Perform, demonstrate & document physical examination that includes general and a detailed neurologic examination as appropriate, based on the history							

Topic 18: Cerebrovascular accident

| S. No. | Name of Activity | Phase Description with Date of Completion | Attempt First (F) Repeat (R) Remedial (Re) | Rating Below Expectation (B) Meet Expectation (M) | Decision of Faculty Completed (C) Not Completed (NC) | Faculty Initial with Date | Feedback Received

Initial of Learner |
|---|---|---|---|---|---|---|---|
| IM 18.6: Distinguish the lesion based on upper vs lower motor neuron, side, site and most probable nature of the lesion | | | | | | | |
| | | | | | | | |
| | | | | | | | |
| | | | | | | | |
| | | | | | | | |
| | | | | | | | |
| | | | | | | | |
| | | | | | | | |

S. No.	Name of Activity	Phase Description with Date of Completion	Attempt First (F) Repeat (R) Remedial (Re)	Rating Below Expectation (B) Meet Expectation (M)	Decision of Faculty Completed (C) Not Completed (NC)	Faculty Initial with Date	Feedback Received Initial of Learner

Topic 18: Cerebrovascular accident

IM 18.7: Describe the clinical features and distinguish, based on clinical examination, the various disorders of speech

Topic 18: Cerebrovascular accident							
S. No.	Name of Activity	Phase Description with Date of Completion	Attempt First (F) Repeat (R) Remedial (Re)	Rating Below Expectation (B) Meet Expectation (M)	Decision of Faculty Completed (C) Not Completed (NC)	Faculty Initial with Date	Feedback Received Initial of Learner
IM 18.10: Choose and interpret the appropriate diagnostic testing in young patients with a cerebrovascular accident (CVA)							

Topic 18: Cerebrovascular accident							
S. No.	Name of Activity	Phase Description with Date of Completion	Attempt First (F) Repeat (R) Remedial (Re)	Rating Below Expectation (B) Meet Expectation (M)	Decision of Faculty Completed (C) Not Completed (NC)	Faculty Initial with Date	Feedback Received Initial of Learner
IM 18.17: Counsel patient and family about the diagnosis and therapy in an empathetic manner							

Topic 19: Movement Disorders

S. No.	Name of Activity	Phase Description with Date of Completion	Attempt First (F) Repeat (R) Remedial (Re)	Rating Below Expectation (B) Meet Expectation (M)	Decision of Faculty Completed (C) Not Completed (NC)	Faculty Initial with Date	Feedback Received Initial of Learner
IM 19.3: Elicit and document and present an appropriate history including onset, progression precipitating and aggravating relieving factors, associated symptoms that help identify the cause of the movement disorders							

S. No.	Name of Activity	Phase Description with Date of Completion	Attempt First (F) Repeat (R) Remedial (Re)	Rating Below Expectation (B) Meet Expectation (M)	Decision of Faculty Completed (C) Not Completed (NC)	Faculty Initial with Date	Feedback Received Initial of Learner
Topic 19: Movement Disorders							
IM 19.4: Perform, demonstrate and document a physical examination that includes a general examination and a detailed neurologic examination using standard movement rating scales							

S. No.	Name of Activity	Phase Description with Date of Completion	Attempt First (F) Repeat (R) Remedial (Re)	Rating Below Expectation (B) Meet Expectation (M)	Decision of Faculty Completed (C) Not Completed (NC)	Faculty Initial with Date	Feedback Received Initial of Learner
Topic 19: Movement Disorders							
IM 19.5: Generate document and present a differential diagnosis and priorities based on the history and physical examination							

S. No.	Name of Activity	Phase Description with Date of Completion	Attempt First (F) Repeat (R) Remedial (Re)	Rating Below Expectation (B) Meet Expectation (M)	Decision of Faculty Completed (C) Not Completed (NC)	Faculty Initial with Date	Feedback Received Initial of Learner
Topic 19: Movement Disorders							
IM 19.6: Make a clinical diagnosis regarding on the anatomical location, nature and cause of the lesion based on the clinical presentation and findings							

	Topic 19: Movement Disorders						
S. No.	Name of Activity	Phase Description with Date of Completion	Attempt First (F) Repeat (R) Remedial (Re)	Rating Below Expectation (B) Meet Expectation (M)	Decision of Faculty Completed (C) Not Completed (NC)	Faculty Initial with Date	Feedback Received Initial of Learner
IM 19.7: Choose and interpret diagnostic and imaging tests in the diagnosis of movement disorders							

Topic 20: Envenomation

S. No.	Name of Activity	Phase Description with Date of Completion	Attempt First (F) Repeat (R) Remedial (Re)	Rating Below Expectation (B) Meet Expectation (M)	Decision of Faculty Completed (C) Not Completed (NC)	Faculty Initial with Date	Feedback Received Initial of Learner
IM 20.2: Describe, demonstrate in a volunteer or a mannequin and educate (to other health care workers / patients) the correct initial management of patient with a snake bite in the field							

S. No.	Name of Activity	Phase Description with Date of Completion	Attempt First (F) Repeat (R) Remedial (Re)	Rating Below Expectation (B) Meet Expectation (M)	Decision of Faculty Completed (C) Not Completed (NC)	Faculty Initial with Date	Feedback Received Initial of Learner
IM 20.4: Elicit and document and present an appropriate history, the circumstance, time, kind of snake, evolution of symptoms in a patient with snake bite							

S. No.	Name of Activity	Phase Description with Date of Completion	Attempt First (F) Repeat (R) Remedial (Re)	Rating Below Expectation (B) Meet Expectation (M)	Decision of Faculty Completed (C) Not Completed (NC)	Faculty Initial with Date	Feedback Received Initial of Learner
Topic 20: Envenomation							
IM 20.5: Perform a systematic examination, document and present a physical examination that includes general examination, local examination, appropriate cardiac and neurologic examination							

S. No.	Name of Activity	Phase Description with Date of Completion	Attempt First (F) Repeat (R) Remedial (Re)	Rating Below Expectation (B) Meet Expectation (M)	Decision of Faculty Completed (C) Not Completed (NC)	Faculty Initial with Date	Feedback Received Initial of Learner
Topic 20: Envenomation							
IM 20.6: Choose and interpret the appropriate diagnostic testing in patients with snake bites							

S. No.	Name of Activity	Phase Description with Date of Completion	Attempt First (F) Repeat (R) Remedial (Re)	Rating Below Expectation (B) Meet Expectation (M)	Decision of Faculty Completed (C) Not Completed (NC)	Faculty Initial with Date	Feedback Received Initial of Learner
	**Topic 21: Poisoning**
	**IM 21.7:** Counsel family members of a patient with suspected poisoning about the clinical and medico legal aspects with empathy

S. No.	Name of Activity	Phase Description with Date of Completion	Attempt First (F) Repeat (R) Remedial (Re)	Rating Below Expectation (B) Meet Expectation (M)	Decision of Faculty Completed (C) Not Completed (NC)	Faculty Initial with Date	Feedback Received Initial of Learner
Topic 22: Mineral, Fluid Electrolyte and Acid base Disorder							
IM 22.13: Identify the underlying acid based disorder based on an ABG report and clinical situation							

S. No.	Name of Activity	Phase Description with Date of Completion	Attempt First (F) Repeat (R) Remedial (Re)	Rating Below Expectation (B) Meet Expectation (M)	Decision of Faculty Completed (C) Not Completed (NC)	Faculty Initial with Date	Feedback Received Initial of Learner
Topic 23: Nutritional and Vitamin Deficiencies							
IM 23.5: Counsel and communicate to patients in a simulated environment with illness on an appropriate balanced diet							

S. No.	Name of Activity	Phase Description with Date of Completion	Attempt First (F) Repeat (R) Remedial (Re)	Rating Below Expectation (B) Meet Expectation (M)	Decision of Faculty Completed (C) Not Completed (NC)	Faculty Initial with Date	Feedback Received Initial of Learner
Topic 24: Geriatrics							
IM 24.2: Perform multidimensional geriatric assessment that includes medical, psycho-social and functional components							

S. No.	Name of Activity	Phase Description with Date of Completion	Attempt First (F) Repeat (R) Remedial (Re)	Rating Below Expectation (B) Meet Expectation (M)	Decision of Faculty Completed (C) Not Completed (NC)	Faculty Initial with Date	Feedback Received Initial of Learner
Topic 25: Infections							
IM 25.4: Elicit document and present a medical history that helps delineate the aetiology of these diseases that includes the evolution and pattern of symptoms, risk factors, exposure through occupation and travel							

Topic 25: Infections							
S. No.	Name of Activity	Phase Description with Date of Completion	Attempt First (F) Repeat (R) Remedial (Re)	Rating Below Expectation (B) Meet Expectation (M)	Decision of Faculty Completed (C) Not Completed (NC)	Faculty Initial with Date	Feedback Received Initial of Learner
IM 25.5: Perform a systematic examination that establishes the diagnosis and severity of presentation that includes: general skin, mucosal and lymph node examination, chest and abdominal examination (including examination of the liver and spleen)							

Topic 25: Infections

S. No.	Name of Activity	Phase Description with Date of Completion	Attempt First (F) Repeat (R) Remedial (Re)	Rating Below Expectation (B) Meet Expectation (M)	Decision of Faculty Completed (C) Not Completed (NC)	Faculty Initial with Date	Feedback Received Initial of Learner
IM 25.6: Generate a differential diagnosis and priorities based on clinical features that help distinguish between infective, inflammatory, malignant and rheumatologic causes							

Topic 25: Infections							
S. No.	Name of Activity	Phase Description with Date of Completion	Attempt First (F) Repeat (R) Remedial (Re)	Rating Below Expectation (B) Meet Expectation (M)	Decision of Faculty Completed (C) Not Completed (NC)	Faculty Initial with Date	Feedback Received Initial of Learner
IM 25.7: Order and interpret diagnostic tests based on the differential diagnosis including: CBC with differential, blood biochemistry, peripheral smear, urinary analysis with sediment, Chest X ray, blood and urine cultures, sputum gram stain and cultures, sputum AFB and cultures, CSF analysis, pleural and body fluid analysis, stool routine and culture and QBC							

S. No.	Name of Activity	Phase Description with Date of Completion	Attempt First (F) Repeat (R) Remedial (Re)	Rating Below Expectation (B) Meet Expectation (M)	Decision of Faculty Completed (C) Not Completed (NC)	Faculty Initial with Date	Feedback Received Initial of Learner
Topic 25: Infections							
IM 25.9: Assist in the collection of blood and other specimen cultures							

Topic 25: Infections

S. No.	Name of Activity	Phase Description with Date of Completion	Attempt First (F) Repeat (R) Remedial (Re)	Rating Below Expectation (B) Meet Expectation (M)	Decision of Faculty Completed (C) Not Completed (NC)	Faculty Initial with Date	Feedback Received Initial of Learner
IM 25.11: Develop an appropriate empiric treatment plan based on the patient's clinical and immune status pending definitive diagnosis							

S. No.	Name of Activity	Phase Description with Date of Completion	Attempt First (F) Repeat (R) Remedial (Re)	Rating Below Expectation (B) Meet Expectation (M)	Decision of Faculty Completed (C) Not Completed (NC)	Faculty Initial with Date	Feedback Received Initial of Learner
Topic 25: Infections							
IM 25.12: Communicate to the patient and family the diagnosis and treatment of identified infection							

S. No.	Name of Activity	Phase Description with Date of Completion	Attempt First (F) Repeat (R) Remedial (Re)	Rating Below Expectation (B) Meet Expectation (M)	Decision of Faculty Completed (C) Not Completed (NC)	Faculty Initial with Date	Feedback Received Initial of Learner

Topic 25: Infections

IM 25.13: Counsel the patient and family on prevention of various infections due to environmental issues

S. No.	Name of Activity	Phase Description with Date of Completion	Attempt First (F) Repeat (R) Remedial (Re)	Rating Below Expectation (B) Meet Expectation (M)	Decision of Faculty Completed (C) Not Completed (NC)	Faculty Initial with Date	Feedback Received Initial of Learner

General Competencies (Show How Level)

	Topic :						
S. No.	Name of Activity	Phase Description with Date of Completion	Attempt First (F) Repeat (R) Remedial (Re)	Rating Below Expectation (B) Meet Expectation (M)	Decision of Faculty Completed (C) Not Completed (NC)	Faculty Initial with Date	Feedback Received Initial of Learner

Topic :							
S. No.	Name of Activity	Phase Description with Date of Completion	Attempt First (F) Repeat (R) Remedial (Re)	Rating Below Expectation (B) Meet Expectation (M)	Decision of Faculty Completed (C) Not Completed (NC)	Faculty Initial with Date	Feedback Received Initial of Learner

General Competencies (Show How Level)

S. No.	Name of Activity	Phase Description with Date of Completion	Attempt First (F) Repeat (R) Remedial (Re)	Rating Below Expectation (B) Meet Expectation (M)	Decision of Faculty Completed (C) Not Completed (NC)	Faculty Initial with Date	Feedback Received Initial of Learner

Topic :							
S. No.	Name of Activity	Phase Description with Date of Completion	Attempt First (F) Repeat (R) Remedial (Re)	Rating Below Expectation (B) Meet Expectation (M)	Decision of Faculty Completed (C) Not Completed (NC)	Faculty Initial with Date	Feedback Received Initial of Learner

SKILL
TRAINING

Certifiable Procedural Skills

A Comprehensive list of skills recommended as desirable for Bachelor of Medicine and Bachelor of Surgery (MBBS)- Indian Medical Graduate (GMER 2019)

S. No.	Procedural Skill	Certified (C) / Not Certified (NC)	Signature of Faculty
1	Venipuncture		
2	Intra-muscular Injection		
3	Intra-dermal Injection		
4	Sub-cutaneous Injection		
5	Intra-venous (IV) Injection		
6	Setting up IV infusion and calculating drip rate		
7	Blood transfusion		
8	Urinary Catheterization		
9	Basic Life Support		
10	Oxygen Therapy		
11	Aerosol Therapy/		

	Nebulization		
12	Ryle's tube insertion		
13	Lumbar Puncture		
14	Pleural and Ascitic aspiration		
15	Cardiac resuscitation		
16	Peripheral Blood Smear interpretation		
17	Bed side urine analysis		
18	Capillary Blood Glucose Testing		
19	Urine Ketone Analysis		

S. No.	Name of Activity	Phase Description with Date of Completion	Attempt First (F) Repeat (R) Remedial (Re)	Rating Below Expectation (B) Meet Expectation (M)	Decision of Faculty Completed (C) Not Completed (NC)	Faculty Initial with Date	Feedback Received Initial of Learner
Procedural Skill:							

Student's descriptive narrative of skill acquired:

S. No.	Name of Activity	Phase Description with Date of Completion	Attempt First (F) Repeat (R) Remedial (Re)	Rating Below Expectation (B) Meet Expectation (M)	Decision of Faculty Completed (C) Not Completed (NC)	Faculty Initial with Date	Feedback Received Initial of Learner
Skill Training							
Procedural Skill:							

Student's descriptive narrative of skill acquired:

		Skill Training					
S. No.	Name of Activity	Phase Description with Date of Completion	Attempt First (F) Repeat (R) Remedial (Re)	Rating Below Expectation (B) Meet Expectation (M)	Decision of Faculty Completed (C) Not Completed (NC)	Faculty Initial with Date	Feedback Received Initial of Learner
Procedural Skill:							

Student's descriptive narrative of skill acquired:

S. No.	Name of Activity	Phase Description with Date of Completion	Attempt First (F) Repeat (R) Remedial (Re)	Rating Below Expectation (B) Meet Expectation (M)	Decision of Faculty Completed (C) Not Completed (NC)	Faculty Initial with Date	Feedback Received Initial of Learner
Skill Training							
Procedural Skill:							

Student's descriptive narrative of skill acquired:

S. No.	**Name of Activity**	**Phase Description with Date of Completion**	**Attempt First (F) Repeat (R) Remedial (Re)**	**Rating Below Expectation (B) Meet Expectation (M)**	**Decision of Faculty Completed (C) Not Completed (NC)**	**Faculty Initial with Date**	**Feedback Received Initial of Learner**
Procedural Skill:							

Skill Training (table title)

Student's descriptive narrative of skill acquired:

Skill Training							
S. No.	Name of Activity	Phase Description with Date of Completion	Attempt First (F) Repeat (R) Remedial (Re)	Rating Below Expectation (B) Meet Expectation (M)	Decision of Faculty Completed (C) Not Completed (NC)	Faculty Initial with Date	Feedback Received Initial of Learner
Procedural Skill:							

Student's descriptive narrative of skill acquired:

Skill Training							
S. No.	Name of Activity	Phase Description with Date of Completion	Attempt First (F) Repeat (R) Remedial (Re)	Rating Below Expectation (B) Meet Expectation (M)	Decision of Faculty Completed (C) Not Completed (NC)	Faculty Initial with Date	Feedback Received Initial of Learner
Procedural Skill:							
Student's descriptive narrative of skill acquired:							

S. No.	Name of Activity	Phase Description with Date of Completion	Attempt First (F) Repeat (R) Remedial (Re)	Rating Below Expectation (B) Meet Expectation (M)	Decision of Faculty Completed (C) Not Completed (NC)	Faculty Initial with Date	Feedback Received Initial of Learner
Skill Training							
Procedural Skill:							

Student's descriptive narrative of skill acquired:

Skill Training							
S. No.	Name of Activity	Phase Description with Date of Completion	Attempt First (F) Repeat (R) Remedial (Re)	Rating Below Expectation (B) Meet Expectation (M)	Decision of Faculty Completed (C) Not Completed (NC)	Faculty Initial with Date	Feedback Received Initial of Learner
Procedural Skill:							
Student's descriptive narrative of skill acquired:							

Skill Training							
S. No.	Name of Activity	Phase Description with Date of Completion	Attempt First (F) Repeat (R) Remedial (Re)	Rating Below Expectation (B) Meet Expectation (M)	Decision of Faculty Completed (C) Not Completed (NC)	Faculty Initial with Date	Feedback Received Initial of Learner
Procedural Skill:							

Student's descriptive narrative of skill acquired:

Skill Training							
S. No.	**Name of Activity**	**Phase Description with Date of Completion**	**Attempt First (F) Repeat (R) Remedial (Re)**	**Rating Below Expectation (B) Meet Expectation (M)**	**Decision of Faculty Completed (C) Not Completed (NC)**	**Faculty Initial with Date**	**Feedback Received Initial of Learner**
Procedural Skill:							
Student's descriptive narrative of skill acquired:							

Skill Training

S. No.	Name of Activity	Phase Description with Date of Completion	Attempt First (F) Repeat (R) Remedial (Re)	Rating Below Expectation (B) Meet Expectation (M)	Decision of Faculty Completed (C) Not Completed (NC)	Faculty Initial with Date	Feedback Received Initial of Learner
Procedural Skill:							

Student's descriptive narrative of skill acquired:

Skill Training

S. No.	Name of Activity	Phase Description with Date of Completion	Attempt First (F) Repeat (R) Remedial (Re)	Rating Below Expectation (B) Meet Expectation (M)	Decision of Faculty Completed (C) Not Completed (NC)	Faculty Initial with Date	Feedback Received Initial of Learner
Procedural Skill:							

Student's descriptive narrative of skill acquired:

Skill Training							
S. No.	Name of Activity	Phase Description with Date of Completion	Attempt First (F) Repeat (R) Remedial (Re)	Rating Below Expectation (B) Meet Expectation (M)	Decision of Faculty Completed (C) Not Completed (NC)	Faculty Initial with Date	Feedback Received Initial of Learner
Procedural Skill:							

Student's descriptive narrative of skill acquired:

S. No.	Name of Activity	Phase Description with Date of Completion	Attempt First (F) Repeat (R) Remedial (Re)	Rating Below Expectation (B) Meet Expectation (M)	Decision of Faculty Completed (C) Not Completed (NC)	Faculty Initial with Date	Feedback Received Initial of Learner
Procedural Skill:							

Skill Training

Student's descriptive narrative of skill acquired:

Skill Training

S. No.	Name of Activity	Phase Description with Date of Completion	Attempt First (F) Repeat (R) Remedial (Re)	Rating Below Expectation (B) Meet Expectation (M)	Decision of Faculty Completed (C) Not Completed (NC)	Faculty Initial with Date	Feedback Received Initial of Learner
Procedural Skill:							

Student's descriptive narrative of skill acquired:

S. No.	Name of Activity	Phase Description with Date of Completion	Attempt First (F) Repeat (R) Remedial (Re)	Rating Below Expectation (B) Meet Expectation (M)	Decision of Faculty Completed (C) Not Completed (NC)	Faculty Initial with Date	Feedback Received Initial of Learner
Skill Training							
Procedural Skill:							

AETCOM MODULE

AETCOM Module No. & Title

AETCOM Competency addressed:

S. No.	Name of Activity	Phase Description with Date of Completion	Attempt First (F) Repeat (R) Remedial (Re)	Rating Below Expectation (B) Meet Expectation (M)	Decision of Faculty Completed (C) Not Completed (NC)	Faculty Initial with Date	Feedback Received Initial of Learner

Student's descriptive narrative of skill acquired:

AETCOM Module No. & Title							
AETCOM Competency addressed:							
S. No.	Name of Activity	Phase Description with Date of Completion	Attempt First (F) Repeat (R) Remedial (Re)	Rating Below Expectation (B) Meet Expectation (M)	Decision of Faculty Completed (C) Not Completed (NC)	Faculty Initial with Date	Feedback Received Initial of Learner

Student's descriptive narrative of skill acquired:

AETCOM Module No. & Title						
AETCOM Competency addressed:						
S. No.	Name of Activity	Phase Description with Date of Completion	Attempt First (F) Repeat (R) Remedial (Re)	Rating Below Expectation (B) Meet Expectation (M)	Decision of Faculty Completed (C) Not Completed (NC)	Faculty Initial with Date	Feedback Received Initial of Learner

Student's descriptive narrative of skill acquired:

AETCOM Module No. & Title							
AETCOM Competency addressed:							
S. No.	Name of Activity	Phase Description with Date of Completion	Attempt First (F) Repeat (R) Remedial (Re)	Rating Below Expectation (B) Meet Expectation (M)	Decision of Faculty Completed (C) Not Completed (NC)	Faculty Initial with Date	Feedback Received Initial of Learner

Student's descriptive narrative of skill acquired:

AETCOM Module No. & Title

AETCOM Competency addressed:

S. No.	Name of Activity	Phase Description with Date of Completion	Attempt First (F) Repeat (R) Remedial (Re)	Rating Below Expectation (B) Meet Expectation (M)	Decision of Faculty Completed (C) Not Completed (NC)	Faculty Initial with Date	Feedback Received Initial of Learner

Student's descriptive narrative of skill acquired:

AETCOM Module No. & Title							
AETCOM Competency addressed:							
S. No.	Name of Activity	Phase Description with Date of Completion	Attempt First (F) Repeat (R) Remedial (Re)	Rating Below Expectation (B) Meet Expectation (M)	Decision of Faculty Completed (C) Not Completed (NC)	Faculty Initial with Date	Feedback Received Initial of Learner

Student's descriptive narrative of skill acquired:

AETCOM Module No. & Title							
AETCOM Competency addressed:							
S. No.	Name of Activity	Phase Description with Date of Completion	Attempt First (F) Repeat (R) Remedial (Re)	Rating Below Expectation (B) Meet Expectation (M)	Decision of Faculty Completed (C) Not Completed (NC)	Faculty Initial with Date	Feedback Received Initial of Learner
Student's descriptive narrative of skill acquired:							

AETCOM Module No. & Title							
AETCOM Competency addressed:							
S. No.	Name of Activity	Phase Description with Date of Completion	Attempt First (F) Repeat (R) Remedial (Re)	Rating Below Expectation (B) Meet Expectation (M)	Decision of Faculty Completed (C) Not Completed (NC)	Faculty Initial with Date	Feedback Received Initial of Learner

Student's descriptive narrative of skill acquired:

PANDEMIC
MODULE

S. No.	Name of Activity	Phase Description with Date of Completion	Attempt First (F) Repeat (R) Remedial (Re)	Rating Below Expectation (B) Meet Expectation (M)	Decision of Faculty Completed (C) Not Completed (NC)	Faculty Initial with Date	Feedback Received Initial of Learner
Pandemic Module							
Competency:							

Student's descriptive narrative of skill acquired:

S. No.	Name of Activity	Phase Description with Date of Completion	Attempt First (F) Repeat (R) Remedial (Re)	Rating Below Expectation (B) Meet Expectation (M)	Decision of Faculty Completed (C) Not Completed (NC)	Faculty Initial with Date	Feedback Received Initial of Learner
Pandemic Module							
Competency:							

Student's descriptive narrative of skill acquired:

Pandemic Module						

S. No.	Name of Activity	Phase Description with Date of Completion	Attempt First (F) Repeat (R) Remedial (Re)	Rating Below Expectation (B) Meet Expectation (M)	Decision of Faculty Completed (C) Not Completed (NC)	Faculty Initial with Date	Feedback Received Initial of Learner
Competency:							

Student's descriptive narrative of skill acquired:

SEMINAR PRESENTATION

		Seminar Presentation				
S. No.	Name of Activity	Phase Description with Date of Presentation	Rating Below Expectation (B) Meet Expectation (M)	Decision of Faculty Completed (C) Not Completed (NC)	Faculty Initial with Date	Feedback Received Initial of Learner

S. No.	Name of Activity	Phase Description with Date of Presentation	Rating Below Expectation (B) Meet Expectation (M)	Decision of Faculty Completed (C) Not Completed (NC)	Faculty Initial with Date	Feedback Received Initial of Learner
Seminar Presentation						

REFLECTIVE WRITING

Reflective Writing
Topic:
What Happened?
So What?
What Next?

Reflective Writing

Topic:

What Happened?

So What?

What Next?

Reflective Writing
Topic:
What Happened?
So What?
What Next?

Reflective Writing

Topic:

What Happened?

So What?

What Next?

Reflective Writing
Topic:
What Happened?
So What?
What Next?

Reflective Writing
Topic:
What Happened?
So What?
What Next?

Reflective Writing
Topic:
What Happened?
So What?
What Next?

Reflective Writing

Topic:

What Happened?

So What?

What Next?

Reflective Writing
Topic:
What Happened?
So What?
What Next?

Reflective Writing
Topic:
What Happened?
So What?
What Next?